The Nervous System

The Nervous System

Circuits of Communication

TORSTAR BOOKS
New York • Toronto

TORSTAR BOOKS INC.
41 Madison Avenue
Suite 2900
New York, NY 10010

THE HUMAN BODY
The Nervous System:
Circuits of Communication

Publisher
Bruce Marshall

Art Director
John Bigg

Creation Coordinator
Harold Bull

Editor
John Clark

Managing Editor
Ruth Binney

Text Commissioning
Hal Robinson

Contributors
Arthur Boylston, Colin Fergusson, Gill
Sales, Peter Sebel, Mike Stoddart,
Safron Whitehead, Phil Whitfield

Text Editors
Wendy Allen, Mike Darton, Martyn
Page, Sandy Shepherd

Researchers
Maria Pal, Jazz Wilson

Picture Researchers
Jan Croot, Kate Duffy, Jessica Johnson,
Dee Robinson

Layout and Visualization
Eric Drewery, Ted McCausland

Artists
Mick Gillah, Aziz Khan, A.W.K.A.
Popkiewicz & Susan Smith, Mick
Saunders

Cover Design
Moonink Communications

Cover Art
Paul Giovanopoulous

Production Director
Barry Baker

Production Coordinator
Janice Storr

Business Coordinator
Candy Lee

Planning Assistant
Avril Essery

International Sales
Barbara Anderson

In conjunction with this series
Torstar Books offers an electronic digital thermometer which
provides accurate body temperature readings in large liquid
crystal numbers within 60
seconds.
For more information write to:
Torstar Books Inc.
41 Madison Avenue
Suite 2900
New York, NY 10010

Marshall Editions, an editorial group that
specializes in the design and publication of
scientific subjects for the general reader,
prepared this book. Marshall has written and
illustrated standard works on technology,
animal behavior, computer usage and the
tropical rain forests which are recommended
for schools and libraries as well as for
popular reference.

Series Consultants

Donald M. Engelman is Professor of
Molecular Biophysics and Biochemistry and
Professor of Biology at Yale. He has
pioneered new methods for understanding
cell membranes and ribosomes, and has also
worked on the problem of atherosclerosis.
He has published widely in professional and
lay journals and lectured at many universities and international conferences. He is
also involved with National Advisory
Groups concerned with Molecular Biology,
Cancer, and the operation of National
Laboratory Facilities.

Stanley Joel Reiser is Professor of
Humanities and Technology in Health Care
at the University of Texas Health Care
Center in Houston. He is the author of
Medicine and the Reign of Technology; coeditor
of *Ethics in Medicine: Historical Perspectives and
Contemporary Concerns;* and coeditor of the
anthology *The Machine at the Bedside.*

Harold C. Slavkin, Professor of
Biochemistry at the University of Southern
California, directs the Graduate Program in
Craniofacial Biology and also serves as Chief
of the Laboratory for Developmental Biology

in the University's Gerontology Center. His
research on the genetic basis of congenital
defects of the head and neck has been
widely published.

Lewis Thomas is Chancellor of the Memorial
Sloan-Kettering Cancer Center in New York
City and University Professor at the State
University of New York, Stony Brook. A
member of the National Academy of
Sciences, Dr. Thomas has served on advisory
councils of the National Institutes of Health.

Consultants for The Nervous System

John J. Caronna is Professor and Vice-
Chairman of the Department of Neurology at
Cornell University Medical College, New
York, and Attending Neurologist at the New
York Hospital. Previously Associate
Professor of Neurology at the University of
California Medical School, San Francisco,
and Associate Editor of *Annals of Neurology,*
he currently serves on various committees,
including a Special Consultancy to the
Editorial Board of the *Journal of Neurology.* He
is the author or coauthor of more than sixty
articles, many concerned with the neurological aspects of brain damage and coma.

Samuel J. Potolicchio is Assistant Professor
at the Georgetown University Medical Center, Washington, DC, where he is also
Director of the University Hospital's Sleep
Disorder Center, EEG Laboratory, and Clinic
for Convulsive Disorders. He has held hospital appointments also in Canada, Switzer-
land and, on a Health Exchange Program, in
the Soviet Union. Much of his hospital work
has concerned EEG analysis and epileptol-

ogy, and his interest in the neuropsychologi-
cal effects of various brain disorders is
reflected in his many publications.

Medical Advisor
Arthur Boylston

© Torstar Books Inc. 1985

**Library of Congress
Cataloging in Publication Data**

The Nervous System: Circuits of
Communication.

   Includes index.
   1. Nervous system. 2. Neurophysiology.
3. Nervous system—Diseases. I. Torstar
Books (Firm) [DNLM: 1. Neurology—
popular works. WL 100 N456]
QP361.N462 1985 612.8 85-13928
ISBN 0-920269-44-3

ISBN 0-920269-22-2 (The Human Body series)
ISBN 0-920269-44-3 (The Nervous System)
ISBN 0-920269-45-1 (leatherbound)
ISBN 0-920269-46-X (school ed.)

20 19 18 17 16 15 14 13 12 11
10   9   8   7   6   5   4   3   2
Printed in Belgium

Contents

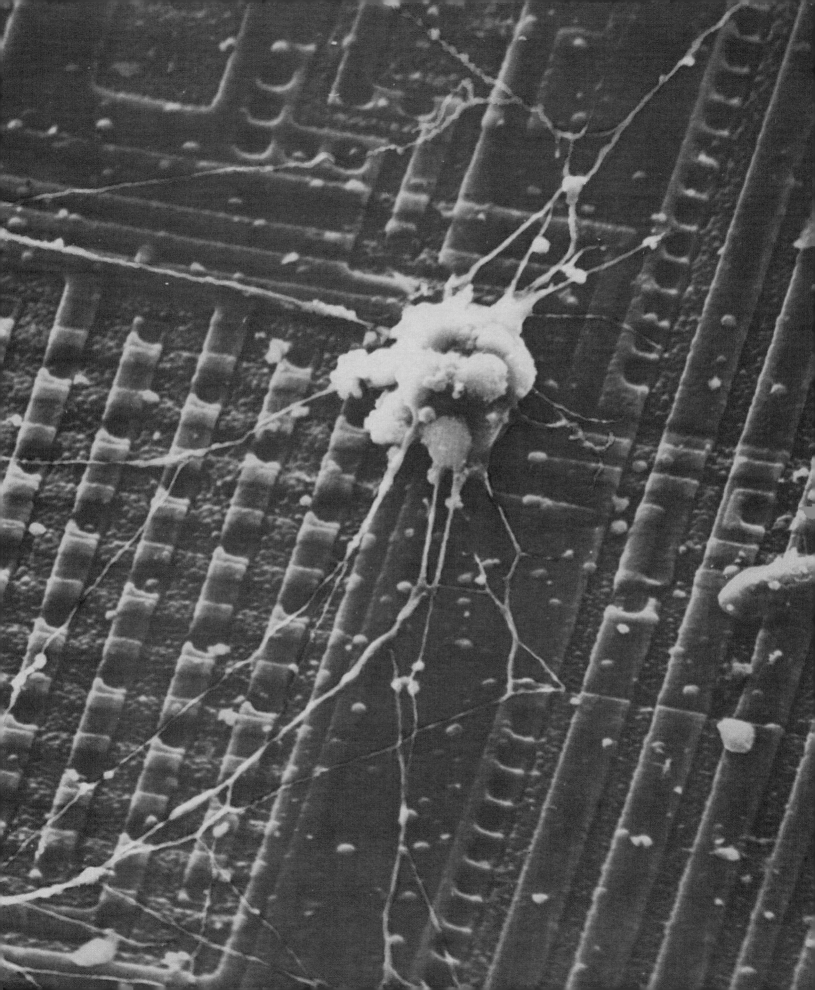

Introduction:

Living on Your Nerves

Trick photography using a scanning electron microscope makes a nerve cell appear to grow on a computer's integrated circuit. Even the most complex man-made circuit cannot begin to match the subtle and intricate circuitry of the human nervous system, although some scientists speculate that "biohybrid" circuits – part living cells, part electronic – may be a future possibility.

Nerves are literally the most sensational aspect of our bodies. While an observer might decree us dead or alive on the strength of a heartbeat or breath, to ourselves "alive-ness" is entirely a matter of what is felt—of the effects of messages nerves deliver to the brain, the brain's lightning analysis, and the resulting actions and sensations.

Of all the body's miraculous components, the nervous system has the distinction of being the most elusive to comprehend. Its complexity and subtlety are likened to futuristic electronic circuitry, yet even the most advanced computer known is primitive by comparison.

With much of its apparatus microscopic and its functioning invisible, the nervous system long resisted attempts to name it, let alone understand it. The term nervous system was not coined until 1665 at a point, historically, when the word nerve was changing its meaning from the "inner fiber" responsible for strength, energy, and courage to a more anatomical definition related to the actual, physical fibers. Nerve and nerves went on to enjoy a multitude of cheerfully conflicting senses—the singular ranging from rudeness to daring, the plural just the opposite.

Figurative meanings aside, the human nervous system consists of two main parts—the central nervous system, comprised of the brain and spinal cord, which interprets information from external sources and coordinates the body's response; and the peripheral nervous system everywhere else in our bodies, which is on a continuous fact-finding mission for the brain. This peripheral system endlessly gathers and transmits data to the central nervous system and then causes the body to act on its orders.

As the fount of all feelings, and of memory and intellect, nerves tell us everything we know about life—tell us that we *are* alive, and that it is no exaggeration to say we live on our nerves.

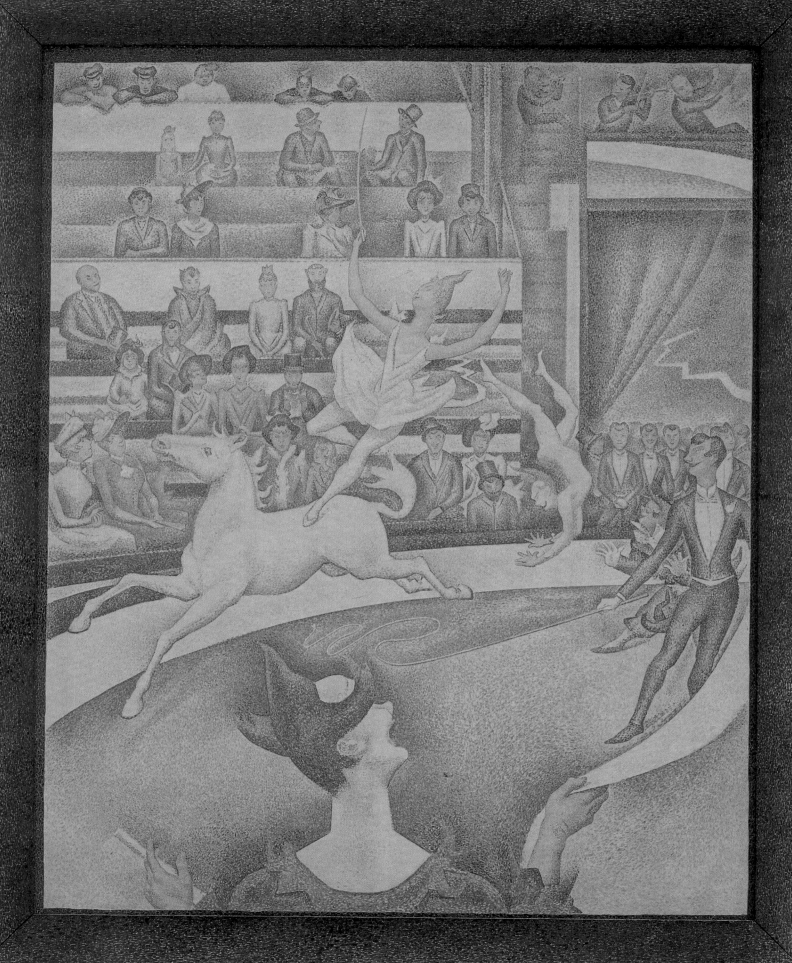

Chapter 1

Mapping the Maze

The human nervous system is the most perfectly-made piece of multifunctional, information-processing "machinery" in the known universe. Whether it is regarded as a divine creation or the product of nearly 4,000 million years of earthly organic evolution (or some intermeshing of the two), the nervous system of *Homo sapiens* is a uniquely complex structure. But this profound conclusion leads to a perplexing philosophical circularity. To collate the necessary information and then to conceive the notion of our nervous system's majesty we must use that selfsame organ system. It is a measure of its awe-inspiring capacities that the system is able to consider itself in this way as an object of attention.

It is almost impossible to demarcate exactly the functions of the different regions of the human nervous system. Those regions are the brain, within the skull; the spinal cord, within the vertebral column of the backbone; and the nerves which lead into and out of the cord. In general terms the coordinating and integrative higher functions involving memory, comparison, and decision-making take place in the brain. The rest of the nervous sytem conveys sensory information to the brain as the "raw material," the data, upon which the brain operates. The nerve tracts of the spinal cord and peripheral nerves also provide the communication system by which the body's movements and reactions are kept finely regulated under control.

When it comes to an analysis of the ultimate components of the physical actions of human beings, a two-part organization becomes apparent. Almost all physical activity can be resolved into a series of individual muscle contractions or secretions by glands. These two fundamental processes are under the control of the spinal nerves. This control constitutes a coordination of activities in what in computer-related language would be termed "real time." Body control is

The bareback rider and acrobat in the French pointillist painter Georges Seurat's Le Cirque *("The Circus") exemplify the perfect coordination needed for many circus acts. Such feats are possible only because men and women possess a highly sophisticated nervous system capable of receiving information, processing it and sending appropriate commands to the body — all in a fraction of a second.*

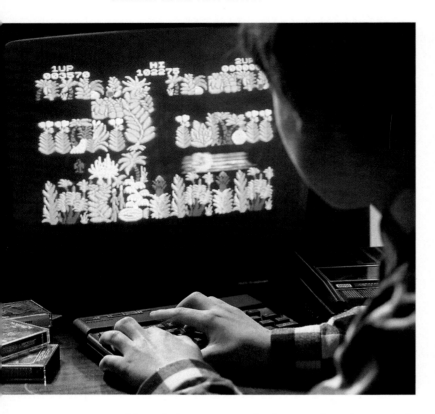

achieved in an unerringly precise, integrated, moment-to-moment fashion.

Patterns of control with longer delays between cause and effect are usually regulated by the body's hormones, which are glandular secretions. The production of these potent chemical messengers, however, usually is itself under some form of nervous control. As a result, immediate bodily responses and longer-term rearrangements of organ functions are intimately intermeshed in one interconnected whole. The essential differences between this pair of control mechanisms are explained by the following examples.

First, consider "real time" rapid control. A young person stands in front of a video game and uses a joystick to manipulate a screen image so as to avoid alien "laser beams." As each beam unpredictably streaks across the screen, an extraordinarily fast pattern of decision-making and consequent muscle activity is taking place. The eyes and the vision-related parts of the central nervous system analyze the image on the screen and transmit the

information along sensory nerves to the brain. Higher brain regions make predictions about the courses of the laser beam, decide on appropriate evasive action and send out nerve impulse messages along motor nerves to the appropriate muscle in the hand and fingers to manipulate the joystick. Before the beam strikes its target, the target has moved. It has moved in time because the whole nervous sytem activity of the player was completed in about a fifth of a second. In the dangers and opportunities of the real rather than the video world, though — as when crossing a busy street — the same staggeringly fast response time of nervous system control is extremely serviceable to us.

Compare this with a second example, an instance of the slower, yet no less vital, pace of hormonal control. A woman's adult reproductive life between puberty and the menopause is controlled by an interweaving pattern of hormonal influences. During this period of 30 to 40 years, except when a child is in the womb, the effect of the hormones is to drive a 28-day cycle of developments in the ovaries and uterus. About one month separates the release of one egg from the release of the next — the same interval occurs between sequential episodes of menstrual bleeding.

The characteristic time intervals associated with the two examples are vastly different. Ovulatory and menstrual cycle: 28 days; video game response time: one-fifth of a second. Events under the influence of one control system are taking place at a rate some 12 million times faster than those of the other. One of the fundamental advantages of having a peripheral nervous sytem is rapid action behavior in response to stimulation from an external source.

Understanding Nerve Function

Nerves conduct nerve impulses to organs. When the impulses arrive at these "end organs" or effectors, they cause activity. The activity is contraction if the effector concerned is a muscle, or it might be the release of digestive enzymes if the end organ is a gland cluster associated with the digestive tract.

This elementary understanding of the nature of nerves and their working has been hard-won.

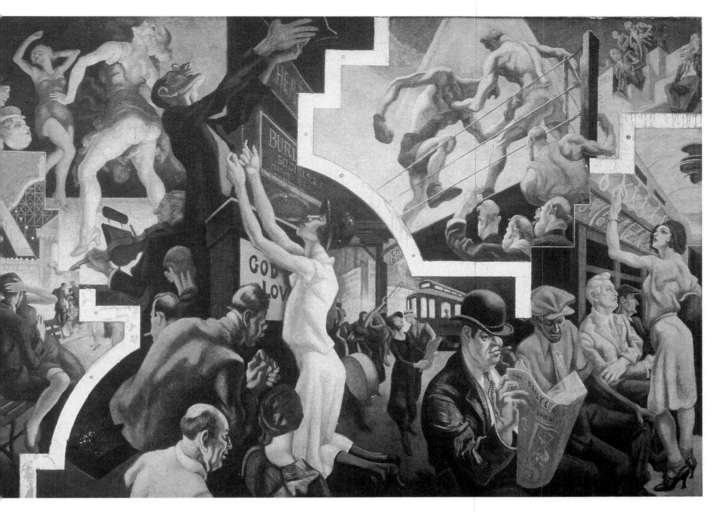

Historically, the nervous system has proved to be one of the most elusive and intractable organ systems to study. There are two main reasons why this should be so.

Firstly, the intrinsic complexity of the tasks performed by the nervous system makes it hard to conceive of a unifying model of its functioning that is not a hopeless distortion of reality. Quite simply, the nervous system as a whole is too complicated for its workings to be understood. At the profoundest level, that is as true today when it is analogized with our most powerful mainframe computers as it was 1,500 years ago when it was still regarded as the pathway for the dispersal of "animal spirits."

The lack of a comprehensive, relevant language for discussing the workings of the nervous system historically has been an enormous hindrance to effective study of that system. If the necessary words, concepts and intellectual "grammar" for the framing of sensible hypotheses about nervous system activity and functioning do not exist, it is exceptionally difficult to perform productive and worthwhile experiments.

This problem was — in part — overcome when it was realized that nerves work in an electrochemical manner. But that understanding and the language and associated insights it spawned were by no means the whole answer to the difficulty. There remains the more fundamental problem of how the basic mechanics of nerve activity relate to the incredibly complex behavior and thoughts that characterize human beings.

The second historically relevant difficulty that slowed developments in this area of understanding might be called the "steam engine and computer" dilemma. It relates to the essentially covert nature of the workings of nerves. They do not operate in ways that mirror any gross, commonsense activities in the world at large. When an impulse passes along a nerve fiber, the fiber does not shorten, change color, emit sounds, move or in any other way change in appearance. This state of affairs can be contrasted with the overt, externally obvious

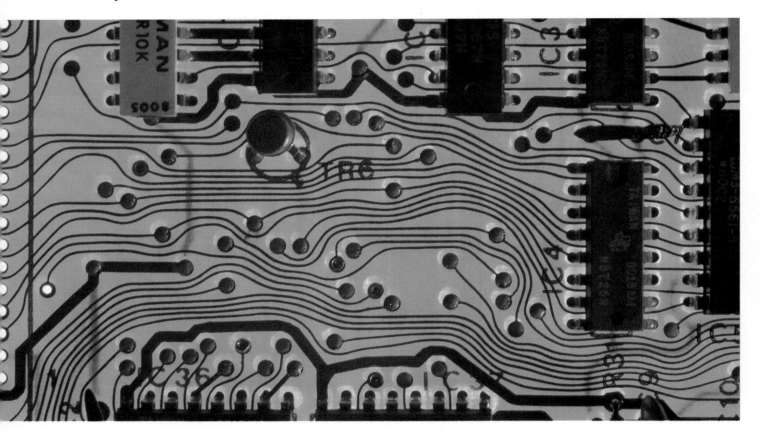

relationship between, say, the contraction of the biceps muscle in the upper arm and the consequent flexing of that limb. The evident causal linkage of muscle shortening and arm bending is equivalent to the steam engine in the "steam engine and computer" analogy. With unaided senses it is possible to work out the basic cycle of an old-fashioned steam engine: expanding steam moves pistons; the pistons move connecting rods; the rods turn the wheels. The cause-and-effect links in this repeating chain of work are externalized and obvious, as are those in the muscular mechanics of bodily movement.

Contrast this situation with a computer. The computer is the classic "black box" as far as the unaided senses of the layman are concerned. If we were to rely for an explanation of a computer's workings only on our sight, touch and hearing, unaugmented by help from machines, a computer might just as well be the result of incantations and

magic. Its actual mode of operation, when running a program, is one of minute, shifting electron flows in microchips — a form of activity invisible and unknowable to man without specialized apparatus. The activity can be directly visualized, for instance, by watching a chip in operation under a scanning electron microscope. The charge differences between conducting and nonconducting parts at each instant show up clearly as differences in the brightness.

Historically, the nervous system has been "the computer" to "the steam engine" of other human organ systems. To a Roman anatomist in the second century A.D. there was absolutely nothing about the structure of a nerve tract that could give clues as to its mode of operation. Only the evidence provided by the traumatic severing of nerves produced a realization that removal of the nervous supply to a region of the body could cause its paralysis or a loss of sensation or both. Nothing at

12

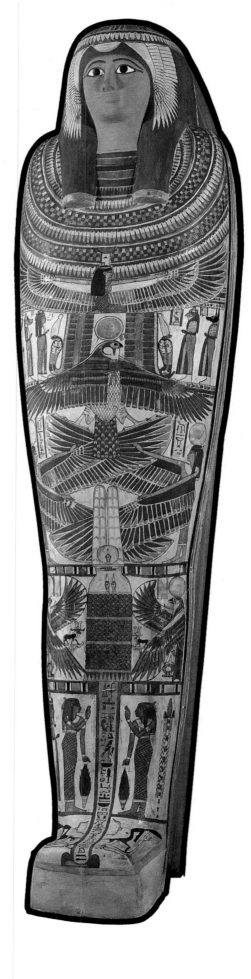

This elaborate mummy case testifies to the importance of funeral practices in ancient Egypt. As a result of the embalming procedures necessary for mummification, basic structures of the nervous system were discovered.

that time could be deduced about the real nature of these effects.

These two problems, namely the sheer enormity of the task carried out by the nervous system and the system's invisible method of working, have conspired in the past to make this collection of tissues the "dark continent" of the body. Infinitely slowly, through insights, guesses, experimentation and sheer good luck, as well as the might of the human intellect, this most impenetrable and uncharted of landscapes of knowledge gave up its secrets. The highpoints of its exploration and mapping over the past 3,000 or more years can give an impression of the arduous work that went into the gathering of each fragment of knowledge.

Ancient Egypt and Greece

The ancient Egyptians knew the basic structures of the brain and the rest of the central nervous system because of the immense emphasis that was placed on the embalming of the dead in their religion. The mummies of the ancient Egyptians are concrete symbols of the fanatical efforts exerted by those peoples to physically preserve their bodies so that their souls might also be preserved. In the course of their complex, highly ritualized embalming procedures, knowledge of the anatomy of the nervous system was — as can be imagined — an inevitable spin-off.

But even the most elaborate of mummification rituals brought the royal embalmers into close contact with only the part of the nervous system in the head. In about 450 B.C. the Greek historian Heroditus described the basic stages of royal mummification in which the first was a removal of the brain from the cranium by means of a hook inserted through the nostrils and by the use of chemicals. It is evident that these techniques could not give a very detailed understanding of the organ systems concerned!

Around 300 B.C. medical understanding took a gigantic leap forward in Alexandria (on the Mediterranean coast of Egypt), which was then one of the administrative and scholastic centers of the Greco-Roman world. At about this time two schools of medical investigation flourished there. The schools are associated with the names of the two foremost investigative physicians of that age —

13

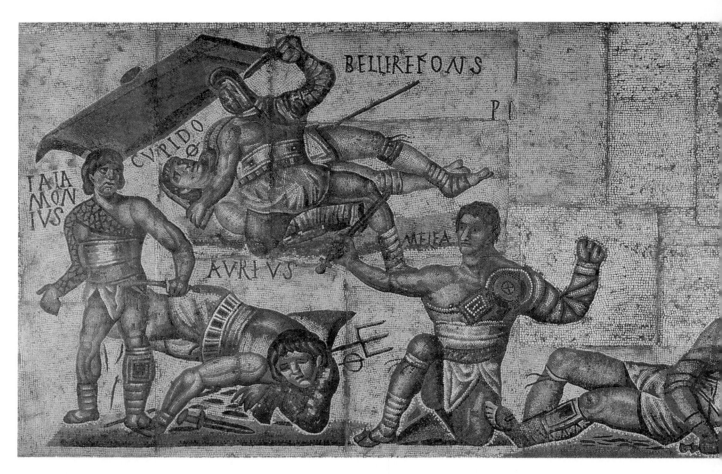

Herophilus and Erasistratos — and both of these searchers after knowledge carried forward our understanding of the nervous system.

Scholars of the history of science have puzzled over the underlying factors which might have been responsible for the blossoming of medical enquiry in Alexandria in the fourth and third centuries B.C. One likely explanation for this crystallization of effort in medical science was the acceptance of human dissections, which were carried out in public and were a natural part of the academic life of the city. It is probable that more than 1,000 years of previous embalming practices had prepared the people to consider such dissections as normal rather than hateful, obscene or blasphemous.

Whatever the root causes of the new attitude, it produced clear advances in understanding the nervous system. It has been said that Herophilus and Erasistratos were, between them, largely responsible for turning the linked areas of anatomy and physiology into areas of real scientific enquiry.

Herophilus, who was born in Chalcedon (now Kadiköy, near the Mediterranean coast of northeastern Turkey) in about 335 B.C., went to Alexandria to teach and practice medicine. Best known as

a pioneering, investigative anatomist, he cast aside the dogma of Aristotle, which held that the heart was the physical location of man's supreme intelligence. Instead, allying himself with the positions of Alcmaeon and Hippocrates, he postulated that the brain was the organizational center of the nervous system. He realized, too, that it was the seat of intelligence.

Herophilus also provided the first written record which demonstrated that spinal sensory nerves have a discrete identity. Earlier workers had realized that numerous elongated structures extend outward from the backbone and the spinal cord within it. But those early studies had scarcely distinguished between the nerves, blood vessels and tendons that make up part of the organic tracery in this region. It took the analytic mind and dissecting skills of Herophilus to show that in the chest and abdominal region, sensory nerves run from the skin to an adjacent portion of the spinal cord and along it make ultimate connections with the brain.

The separate identity of the motor nerves arising from the spinal cord was verified by Erasistratos. The founder of the second Alexandrian school of

14

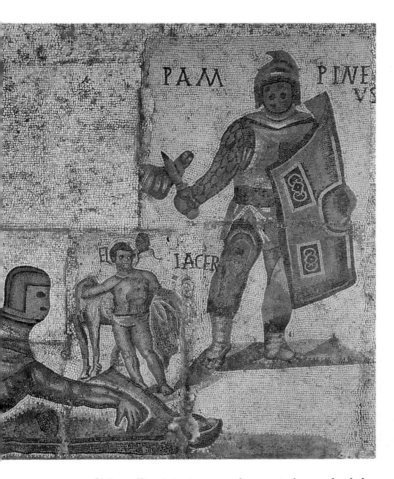

Treating the injuries sustained in
gladiatorial contests enabled the
Roman physician Galen to make
many discoveries about the nervous
system, including the relation of
nerve damage to specific symptoms.

Galen: The Father of Medicine

Emerging from this background in the second century A.D., however, was a personality of such perception and industry that he is well placed to be called the most accomplished physician of the last 2,000 years. Galen, born in Pergamos in A.D. 129 or 130, was fated to travel along the roads of medicine. In his own writings he explained that when he was aged 17 his father, an architect, was visited in a dream by Asclepius (the Greek god of medicine), who told him to allow his son to be instructed in the ways of a physician. The god's order was obeyed and Galen, in the manner of those days, journeyed from one medical center to another to learn from the great teachers of the time.

Galen finished his medical training in Alexandria, then returned to his home city and spent four years as a physician in the College of Gladiators. In about A.D. 160 he traveled to Rome and rapidly established himself as the foremost medical man of his day. Over the next 40 years until his death in A.D. 200 he was an astoundingly prolific writer on medicine.

By direct observation with dissections of human cadavers and various animals, Galen produced a vast amount of high-quality information on human anatomy, pathology and physiology. Some of his concepts of physiology, however, were encumbered with erroneous ideas that could be traced back to Erasistratos. These included the idea that the blood was made in the liver from chyle (the fatty, milklike fluid found in the lymphatic system) and "pneuma" the spirit or essence of air.

The physiology of the nervous system believed by Galen was embedded inextricably in this distorted framework of ideas. In particular, blood was known to be carried by arteries to the brain but was thought to be importantly altered there. Its new manifestation was psychic "pneuma," regarded as a mysterious fluid "animal spirit" which was thought to pass along the nerves to all parts of the body.

Given the constraints under which Galen was working, this idea bears a remarkable resemblance to modern ideas. If "nerve impulse" is read for "animal spirit," a description is derived which is not far removed from one that modern minds would find acceptable. Because of the authority of

medicine, Erasistratos was born at the end of the fourth century B.C. on the island of Cos in the Aegean. After much study and travel in mainland Greece he finally settled in Alexandria. He deduced from dissections that discrete nerves lead out from the spinal cord to specific regional groups of body muscles. These nerve tracts are the motor nerves, the activities of which stimulate muscles to contract. With the realization that each region of the body has separate sensory and motor nerve supplies, the anatomical foundation for much of the next 2,000 years' worth of neurological investigation had been laid.

During the second century B.C. the focus of scientific and cultural activities in the Mediterranean world shifted from the eastern Hellenic region to the Roman center. Greek physicians and those trained in the several Greek schools of medical theory homed in on the lucrative market provided by the rich elite of Roman society. With an emphasis on practical methods of treatment rather than investigative efforts, this shift of the center of the medical world did little to encourage new research or even to increase the overall availability of fundamental knowledge.

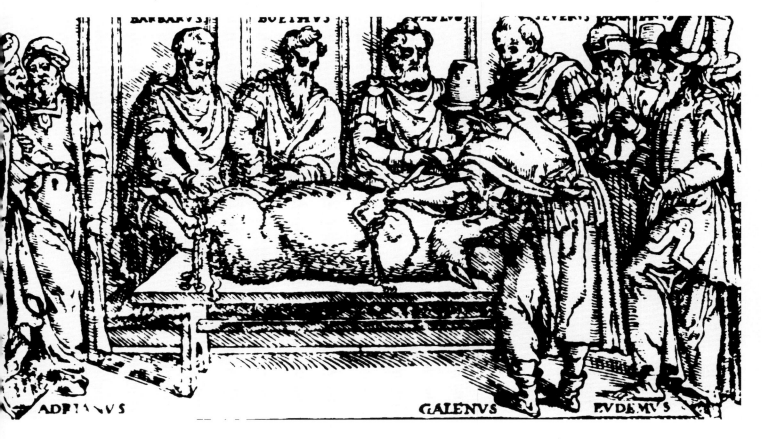

ADRIANVS   GALENVS   EVDEMVS

Galen in early medicine, the animal spirit dogma was believed in some form or another through most of the Middle Ages.

Despite Galen's conceptual shortcomings, his direct observational work on the human nervous system was of exceptional quality. As a superb anatomist he made remarkable advances in the understanding or the organization of the cranial nerves, which emerge from the base of the brain. He recognized seven of the twelve pairs, and made further discoveries concerning the cervical nerves (the spinal nerves in the neck), nerve ganglia (groups of nerve cells outside the brain and spinal cord) in general, and a portion of the sympathetic nervous system (which controls some involuntary body functions).

Galen's ultimate achievement in the area of nervous mechanisms was, however, one of correlation. Through his many observations of human injuries — which his position as physician to gladiators enabled him to make — he came to understand the links between injury or disease in particular parts of the peripheral nervous system and specific symptoms. Thus he could begin, for instance, to link paralysis of particular muscles in a specific part of the body with precisely localized damage to nerve tracts or the spinal cord.

This level of understanding, achieved some 1,800 years ago, is in itself a remarkable tribute to the energy, perspicacity and intelligence of this man. It comes as a shock from a twentieth-century vantage point to link Galen's achievement with his surroundings. In an age when gladiators were fighting to the death in the amphitheater, a physician tending their wounds had mastered some of the central mysteries of the wiring circuitry of the human nervous system. What is more he had achieved this with little more than a sharp knife, sharp eyes and an even sharper intellect.

At the time of Galen's death in about A.D. 200, the

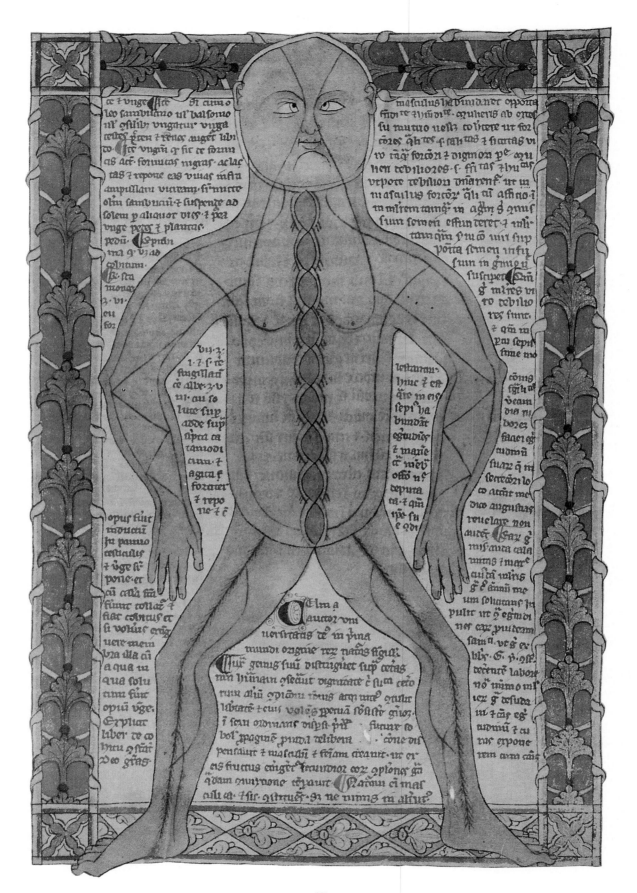

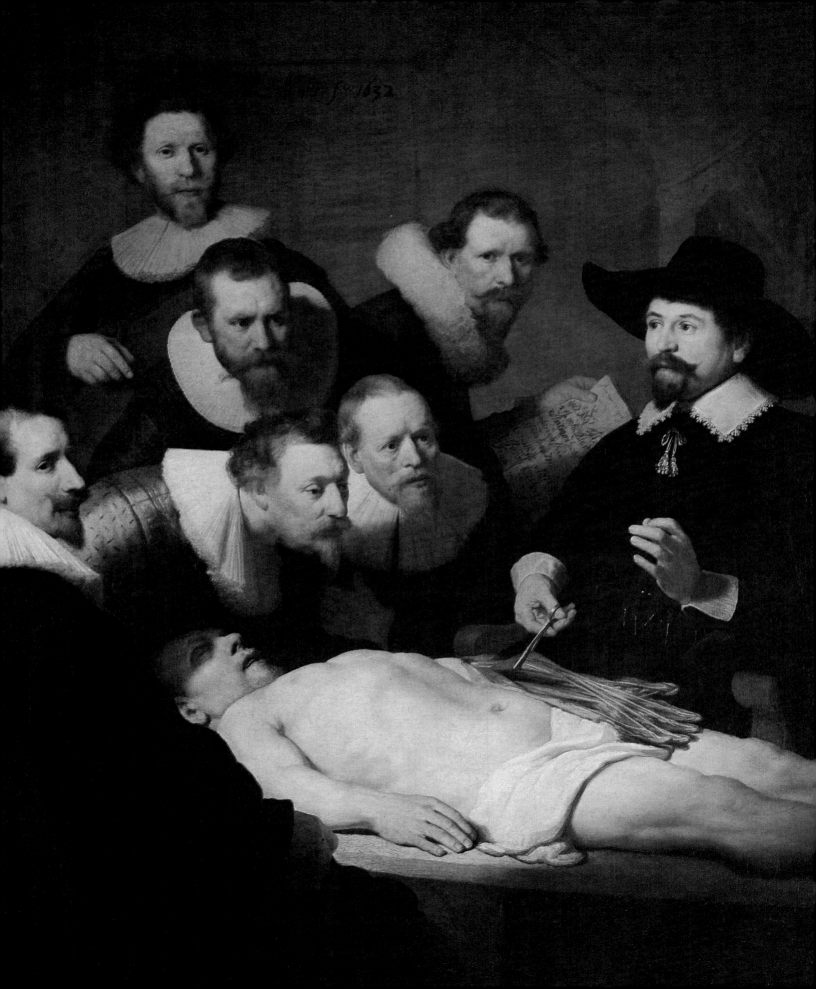

The Anatomy Lesson of Dr Tulp *by Rembrandt illustrates the importance of human dissection to medicine. During the Renaissance, dissection of cadavers led to many discoveries about the nervous system.*

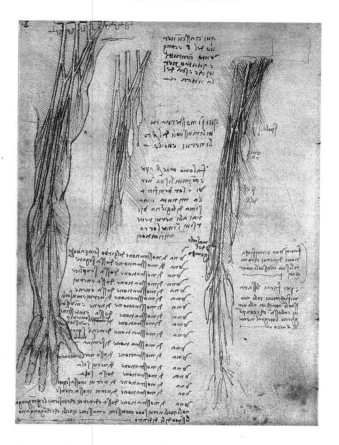

Leonardo da Vinci, probably the most famous thinker of the Renaissance, made accurate sketches of his many human dissections. One of his drawings of the nerves in the arm is shown below.

Roman Empire was, however, only about 270 years away from its final overthrow by the barbarians. Waves of peoples from the east and north brought an end to the network of civilization and society that could engender and then foster a medical mind and a medical life like Galen's. This tremendous upheaval created an enormous hiatus in the flow of European history and marked the beginning of the Dark Ages. As Lawrence Durrell so poignantly crystallizes it in his book *Prospero's Cell*: "It was an Ice Age settling down on the Roman Empire and . . . it could not be averted or withstood."

Unavertable and unwithstandable, the new barbarians came. The Empire was shattered and almost all scientific enquiry of any sort was at an end. Classical ideas were salvaged from the fifth to the tenth centuries A.D. by a few monks who gathered together remnants of older texts. But the most direct inheritors of the flame of Hellenic and Roman scientific thought were the Arabic scholars of the Middle East. They recognized the value of the classical texts. Not only did they preserve them, they continued investigative, experimental science. Without their endeavors, the scientific Renaissance when it finally came to Europe like a long-delayed birth, would have been a sickly infant indeed.

Renaissance Discoveries

It is possible to focus on a series of specific discoveries in neurological science made during the Renaissance which began to fill out the basic picture provided by Galen centuries before. In about 1540 Vesalius, another skillful anatomist and dissector, removed the nerve sheaths of nerve bundles, stimulated nerves by contact and produced reactions in the muscles to which they were connected. In 1552 Eustachius — after whom is named the eustachian tube (linking the cavity of the middle ear to the nasopharynx) — produced marvelous engravings of the human brain and nervous system, including a remarkably accurate portrayal of the sympathetic nerves. But his nerve engravings, although of stunningly high fidelity to the anatomical reality, played little part in the onward movement of knowledge in his own time, principally because publication of his work was delayed until 1714. Meanwhile in the 1660s the Italian physiologist Marcello Malpighi, with the benefit of

the newly-invented microscope, had recognized sensory nerve endings for the first time.

From the mid-seventeenth century to the beginning of the nineteenth there were a series of overlapping insights into the subject of nerve action. Much of this advance was concerned with nerve-muscle interactions.

In his book published in 1664 *Description du corps humain* ("Description of the Human Body") the French philosopher and investigator René Descartes demonstrated that he already understood some of the essential features of what we would call a reflex action. He described such an action in the language of his age — in relation to the soul. The core of his argument was that when an organ of the human body tends toward a particular action there is no need of a soul to instigate that action. It may be presumed that in this context he was using the idea of soul in the sense of conscious will or thought. The involuntary con-

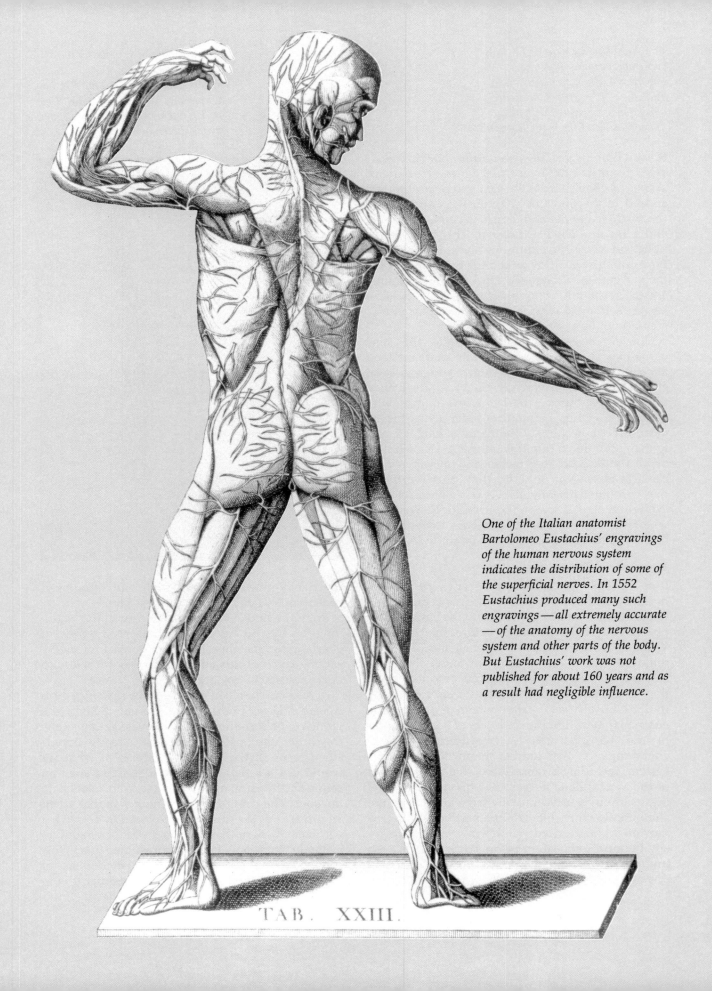

One of the Italian anatomist
Bartolomeo Eustachius' engravings
of the human nervous system
indicates the distribution of some of
the superficial nerves. In 1552
Eustachius produced many such
engravings—all extremely accurate
—of the anatomy of the nervous
system and other parts of the body.
But Eustachius' work was not
published for about 160 years and as
a result had negligible influence.

TAB. XXIII.

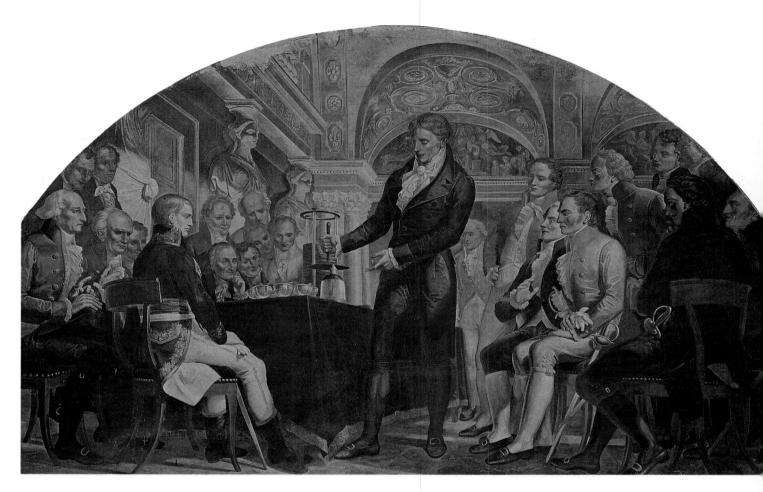

striction of the pupil of the eye when exposed to bright light — the pupillary reflex as it is known — was one of the examples that led him to this conclusion about reflex actions.

Robert Whytt (1717–1766), an Englishman, disagreed with the mechanistic world view of Descartes. He considered reflexes to involve a linkage of sensory stimuli with a receptive and organizing soul. But he did understand the vital role that the spinal cord rather than the brain plays in establishing many reflex actions. The studies that led him to this conclusion related to frogs that had been decapitated. When the leg of a headless frog is pricked with a sharp instrument, the leg jerks. It does so because of the intact linkage of sensory nerves from the skin of the leg to the spinal cord — appropriate nervous connections within the cord and outgoing reflex motor connections to the muscles of the leg — the reflex loop. These early experiments showed that if the nerve connections between the leg and the spinal cord are cut, the response of the leg muscles to skin pricking is also abolished. Whytt had the perspicacity to realize the underlying importance of this simple experiment.

The Italian physicist Alessandro Volta demonstrates his "voltaic pile," the first electric battery. In the late eighteenth century there was much dispute about the nature of electricity. Luigi Galvani, from his experiments on frogs, thought that animal tissue was necessary to produce a current. Volta maintained that it could be generated using metals alone. Volta was proved correct with his completion of the electric battery in 1800. But although Galvani was wrong about the nature of electricity, his experiments demonstrated the electrochemical basis of the working of nerves — an important step.

Luigi Galvani

Advocate of "Animal Electricity"

"Galvanometer" and "galvanizing" are both terms derived from the surname of Luigi Galvani, the renowned Italian anatomist although, in fact, he invented neither the instrument nor the process. Successive scientists regarded him so highly that they gave his name to developments achieved after his death.

He was born on September 9, 1737 in Bologna, the third child of a well-to-do family. He originally studied theology but transferred to philosophy and medicine at Bologna University. This institution had a long history of anatomical research and Galvani quickly became interested in the subject. By the age of 25 he was already a lecturer in anatomy at the university and an instructor at the affiliated Institute of Science.

In 1762 he married Lucia, the only daughter of a distinguished anatomist Professor Galeazzi, and she was to help him in many of his experiments. He is recorded as having been a kind-hearted man and often treated those who could not afford to pay.

In the 1770s, after making important observations on the hearing of birds and functioning of the kidneys, Galvani began to experiment with the possibilities of muscle

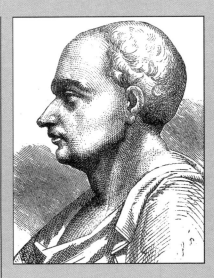

stimulation using electricity. He placed skinned frogs on a table close to an electric machine or condenser (such as a Leyden jar) and noticed that when the machine was activated the muscles of the frog twitched. He observed that the same thing happened when frogs were laid out on metal during a thunderstorm and no electric machine was present. He also hung dissected frogs from copper hooks fastened to iron railings outside his study and discovered that by pressing the hook through the frog's spinal column against the railing, muscular contractions occurred. More simply, two metals together seemed to produce similar results.

Galvani stated "these results surprised us greatly and led us to suspect that the electricity was inherent in the animal itself." He concluded that animal tissue contained an innate force called "animal electricity."

Alessandro Volta, a leading physicist, quickly disputed his conclusions. Thereafter began a professional rivalry dividing the scientific world into those who supported Galvani's "animal electricity" and those who supported Volta's so-called "metallic electricity" believing the force to be inherent in the metal. Personally the two men greatly respected each other and Volta wrote of Galvani's research "it contains one of the most beautiful and surprising discoveries, and the germ of several others."

In later life Galvani was dispirited, not least by the general acceptance of Volta's theories but also by the death of his wife to whom he was greatly attached. When the newly established Cisalpine Republic made a ruling that teaching staff should swear an oath of allegiance to the state, Galvani refused and was dismissed. His job was finally offered back to him but by this time he was an old man. He died (in the house in which he was born) on December 4, 1798.

The Italian scientist Luigi Galvani made the famous discovery that frogs' legs could be made to twitch by touching them with different metals. To investigate, he performed countless similar experiments —

some of which are illustrated in the engraving. He eventually concluded (wrongly, it is now known) that a special type of fluid "animal electricity" flowed from the brain through the nerves to muscles.

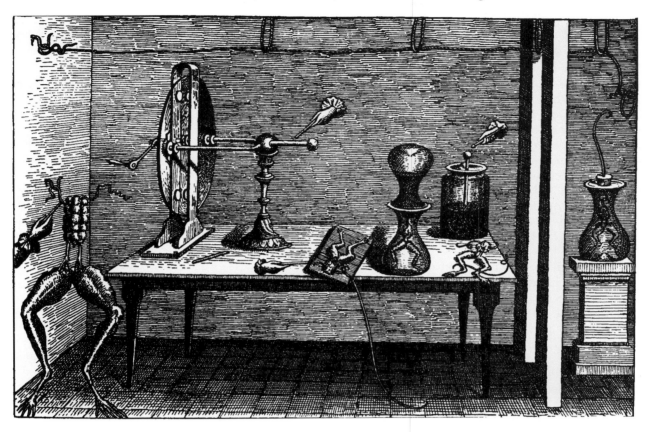

From Frogs to Modern Theories

The humble frog also plays two other center-stage roles in the drama of the understanding of human nervous activity. The roles were not acted out at the same time nor in the same geographical theater. Act I occurred in Italy in about 1780. The curtain rose on Act II in Berlin, Germany, during the first years of the nineteenth century.

The Italian example is the momentous breakthrough made by Luigi Galvani about twenty years before the beginning of the nineteenth century. He was intrigued by the possible role of electricity in a variety of living things. His interest was initially fueled by earlier findings. In 1772 it had been shown that one of the electric fish of the genus *Torpedo* produces massive electric shocks. It utilizes these electrical discharges to stun its prey and to protect itself from predators. Other workers had used the Leyden jar (a primitive device for storing electric charge) to investigate the effect of electrical

discharges on hearts and muscles. Indeed, demonstrations of the power and properties of the electrical spark were of consuming interest throughout the eighteenth century. One of the best known of these demonstrations is Benjamin Franklin's kite experiment of 1752, in which he showed that lightning is electric by flying a kite in a thunderstorm. (It was he who popularized the terms "positive" and "negative.")

Galvani's interests and purposes were more subtle and biologically oriented. He was an eminent doctor of Bologna, where he was born in 1737 and died in 1798. His findings have become such an important strand in the rich fabric of physiological science that it has become difficult to disentangle fact, myth and anecdote concerning the manner of his discoveries. One version is that, in the year 1790, Galvani had skinned some frogs to make broth for his wife, who was ill. A knife which had been placed beside an electric machine became charged and when it touched a frog's leg, the leg began to kick.

Whatever the true stimulus for investigation, Luigi Galvani began to look at the effects of electric sparks on the muscles of frogs' legs. In the course of these studies he became aware that muscles could be made to contract when brought into contact with strips of different types of metal. What he had inadvertently discovered was that the tiny electrical currents that are set up when dissimilar metals touch could efficiently stimulate nerves and muscles. He had discovered the electrochemical basis of the workings of nerves, and from then on investigations on nerves were correctly focused. The modern science of electrophysiology was thus instituted.

But the birth brought much controversy. Galvani thought that his experiments showed evidence of an animal electricity residue in tissues. This view was disputed by other scientists, including the famous Italian physicist Alessandro Volta. So some 200 years ago the men who gave their names to the galvanometer and the volt were intellectually struggling with each other and with the formative concepts of electrophysiology.

The second frog-based demonstration of vital importance to neurology and neurophysiology was a historic experiment carried out by the German physiologist Johannes Müller in about 1830. Müller's knowledge was great and varied; he was one of the founders of the science of comparative physiology and he also made far-reaching discoveries over a wide range of other life science disciplines, including marine biology, physiology, anatomy and developmental embryology. As part of his contribution to neurophysiology he developed the concept of "specific nerve energies." This suggested that the sensory nerves from each type of sense organ — that is, the nerves that carry information from the sense organ toward the central nervous system — directly determine the type of sensory stimulation experienced, irrespective of the manner in which the nerve itself was stimulated.

An extraordinarily able experimentalist, Müller was nonetheless a "vitalist." He believed that living organisms possessed a transcendental "vital force" that differentiated the living from the inanimate.

He extended this conviction to one area of nervous behavior, considering that the impulse carried by a nerve was a manifestation of the vital force and so could not be directly investigated. In particular he held that its speed could not be determined experimentally. But he was proved wrong only ten years after this pronouncement when one of his pupils, the famous German scientist Hermann von Helmholtz, successfully measured the speed of a nerve impulse through a series of experiments again using a frog. First he stimulated a nerve connected to a muscle at a point on the nerve that was close to the muscle; then he stimulated the nerve at a point farther down, and managed to measure the additional time the muscle took to respond. It was also Helmholtz's contention that the vitalist case was not consistent with the law of conservation of energy.

Müller himself used a frog preparation for a characteristically elegant demonstration of spinal nerve function. He categorically illustrated the different roles of the posterior (dorsal) and anterior (ventral) roots or nerve tracts that are the separated components of each spinal nerve. The idea that the posterior roots are the sensory nerve tracts whereas the anterior ones contain motor nerves going from the central nervous system toward the muscles is credited to Sir Charles Bell in England in 1811. The French scientist François Magendie provided some experimental corroboration of this scheme in 1822, but it was left to Müller in 1830 to confirm the truth of the idea.

The posterior spinal nerves of a frog have relatively thick and long roots which extend a long way posteriorly before fusing. Müller took advantage of this fortuitous configuration. When he cut a posterior root next to its insertion in the spinal cord and then stimulated the root with forceps, no muscle contraction occurred. When the same procedure was carried out on intact or severed anterior roots, vigorous muscle contractions took place.

With the findings of Bell, Magendie, Müller and Helmholtz the world entered the modern era of scientific study of a nervous system. The way was clear for the explosion of knowledge which has occurred in the subsequent century and a half, and which is described in the following chapters.

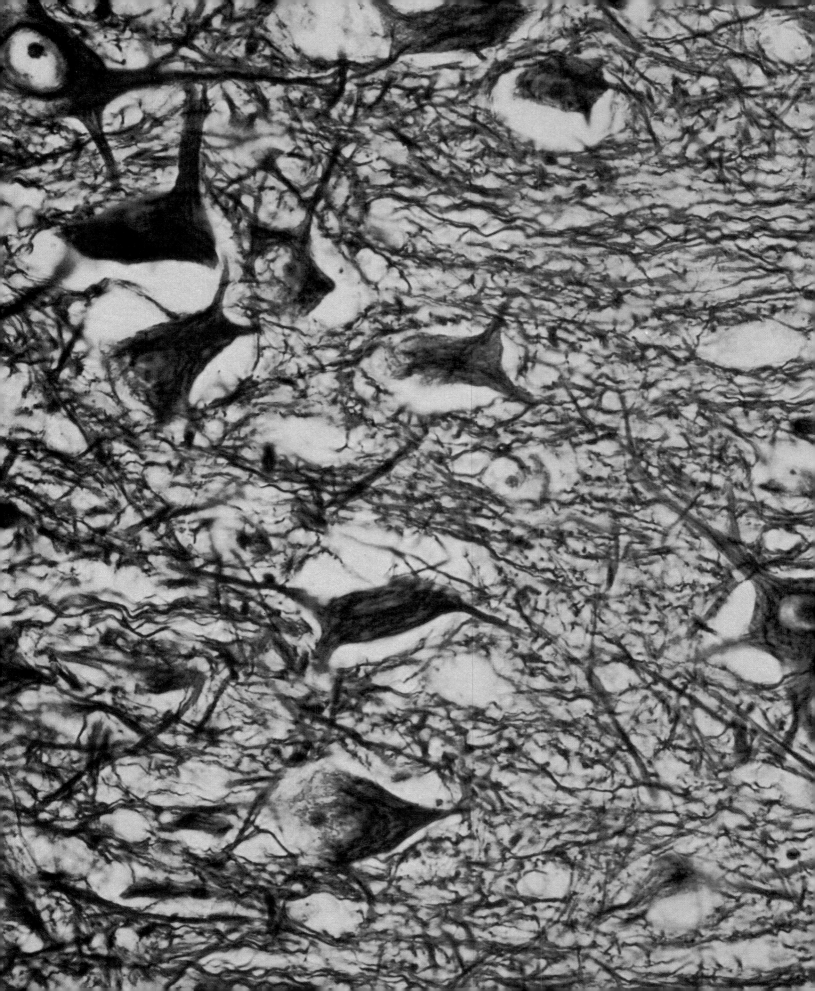

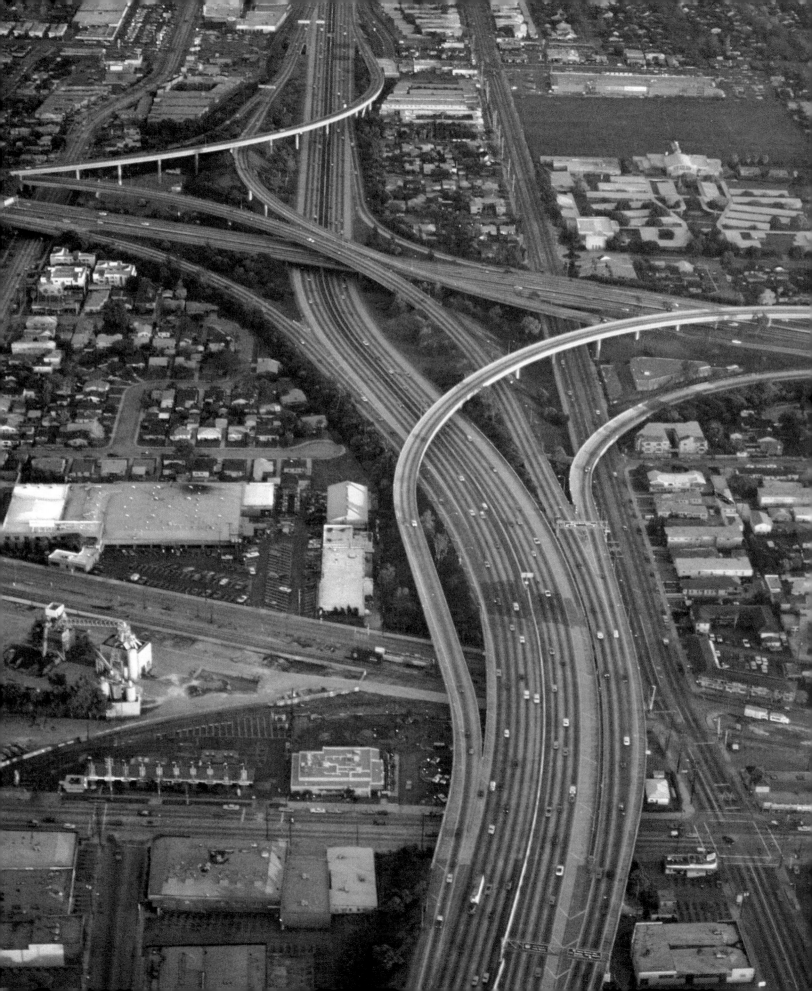

Chapter 2

Simplicity to Sophistication

Many things that men and women do – such as climbing up a dangerous rock face, or driving fast in a Grand Prix – require great nerve. Other activities require intense and precise control, such as playing a musical instrument to concert standard, or dancing a solo in *Sleeping Beauty*. A sea anemone or a starfish is extremely unlikely ever to be able to emulate such feats, not simply because it does not have the right number of arms, legs, hands and fingers but because it lacks a nervous system in any way complex enough for it.

It is not just the human brain which is highly developed, but also the central and peripheral nervous system. Hidden within the bony yet flexible tube of the spine lies the great arterial freeway of the central nervous system, branching out over all its length toward every part of the body in a network of nervous highways and byways. Nerves reach every extremity of the body, from the tips of the toes and fingers to the top of the scalp, as well as to the central organs of heart, liver, lungs and gut. In this way neurophysiologists can regard the human body as a highly sophisticated electronic box in which tiny currents flow this way and that to carry out the dictates of the brain and the sense organs. An overview of this amazing vital system logically begins, therefore, with an examination of the way in which it is structured.

What is the Nervous System?

Nerves are single cells which have become specialized for carrying information from one part of the body to another. Usually a great number lie together, rather like the individual fibers in a rope or cable, and form a nerve cord. When people speak of nerves it is usually nerve cords that they mean, for a single nerve cell may be as small as four-thousandths of a millimeter (4 microns) thick — many times thinner than a hair.

In the living animal nerves appear creamy white

Just as millions of people daily speed along the complex network of interweaving highways to reach their destinations, so the brain despatches and receives messages along a multitude of nerve routes. Nerves spread out to the most distant parts of the body sending controlling messages to the body's organs and passing sensory information back to the brain.

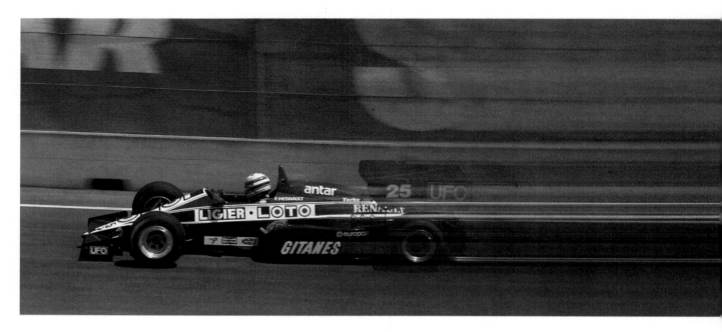

in color, although the color appears to fade somewhat as the bundles split up into ever more tiny fragments. Each nerve cell has the same basic structure as every other cell in the body; there is a nucleus with its contained microstructures and various subcellular inclusions or organelles. But the nerve cell is differentiated from other cells by having a tuft of short, rootlike projections at one end of the cell body called "dendrites," and a long, thin, projection from the other called the "axon." Although they may be extremely thin, nerve cells are sometimes astonishingly long. The nerve from the base of the spine to the tip of the toe in an average human is about three feet in length, and that running from the shoulder to the front hoof of a giraffe may be almost six feet in length. The tip of the axon may subdivide up to 150 times and attach to 150 separate muscle fibers. Not all axons are this length however, and many are only a fraction of an inch long.

Most axons do not end directly in a block of muscle. Most are only a single link in a long chain of nerve cells, each axon making near contact with the dendrites of the next cell. A tiny gap or "synapse" is left between cells, and each nerve impulse has to jump across this gap. Although the synapse is minute – perhaps as little as

1/100,000mm (0.1 micron) – it is too large for a wave of electricity to cross. At its very tip the axon has a number of tiny secretory cups, or vesicles, which produce a trace of a special chemical substance known as a "neurotransmitter" when the electrical wave reaches them. Neurotransmitters then diffuse across the synapse and excite the dendrites of the next cell to induce a new electrical wave in their cell, and so on down the chain. Each synapse offers a certain amount of resistance to the passage of the nervous message, which gradually becomes less strong the farther it travels from its origin.

Why the gaps? Part of the answer seems to be to permit more than just one cell to influence the next. Most nerve cells receive their stimulation from more than one cell higher up the line, and so receive more than just one kind of information. Some of the contributing cells may have an inhibitory effect; others stimulate the cell. In this way the nerve impulse is subject to many different, and at times opposing, influences. Connections of this sort integrate and organize the nerve paths, and permit the great sensitivity in precision and control which typifies the highest vertebrates, and the mammals in particular.

In much the same way as a thick electrical cable offers less resistance to the flow of electricity than

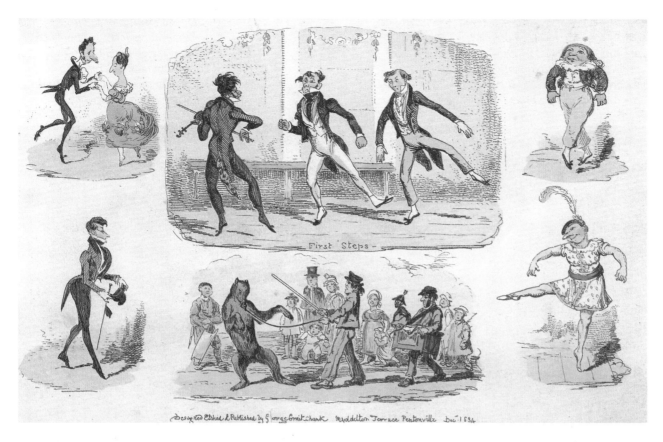

First Steps

Designed Etched & Published by George Cruikshank Myddelton Terrace Pentonville Dec 1834

a thin wire, so nerve impulses travel faster in thick axons than in thin ones. But thick axons would not be suitable in small vertebrates such as field mice or minnows, for the nervous system is only one of several systems which must be fitted into the living body. Yet these small creatures are often extremely active, so how is the problem overcome? The white color of nerves is not actually the color of the nerve cell but of a fatty sheath which envelops the axon, and this structure enables impulses to pass with great speed. The fatty substance is called "myelin;" nerves with this sheath are therefore described as "myelinated," and those without it are known as "unmyelinated."

Nerve impulses can flow only from the axon of one cell to the dendrite of another, and never in the opposite direction.

When you wish to walk, impulses travel from your brain via your central nervous system and outward toward the muscles of your legs and feet. The nerves which carry these instructions are known as "motor neurons," because they trigger some motor (movement) activity. They are also known as "efferent" fibers because they transmit information only away from the central nervous system. But if you should happen to put your foot down on a thumbtack, a different set of nerves or neurons conveys the anguished message back to the central nervous system. These sensory neurons originate in the peripheral sense organs and send their message in the opposite direction to that of the motor neurons. They are termed "afferent," because their information travels toward the spine.

Both motor and sensory nerves may run in the same nerve cord, and superficially look the same as one another. In reality, though, each carries information in one direction only.

So far the nervous system has been considered only as the tool of voluntary will. But much of the human body is not under voluntary control. There is no way of voluntarily controlling, say, kidney function, heart rate, digestion, or menstruation. Yet all these functions, and a great many more, are controlled and integrated by the various parts of the nervous system.

The part of the system responsible for involuntary control is known as the "autonomic" nervous system. Anatomists and physiologists divide the autonomic nervous system into two sections, the "sympathetic" system, in which neurons originate from the spinal column, and the "parasympathetic" system, in which neurons originate from the base of the brain. Sympathetic

The abundance of sensory receptors in the fingertips enables a person to read Braille (below), which is a code of raised dots, The information received is instantly passed by nerve cells (bottom) to the brain.

Branched endings of axons, terminating in small swellings called boutons, synapse on the large cell body of a neuron. Terminal boutons release the chemical that transmits impulses across the synapse.

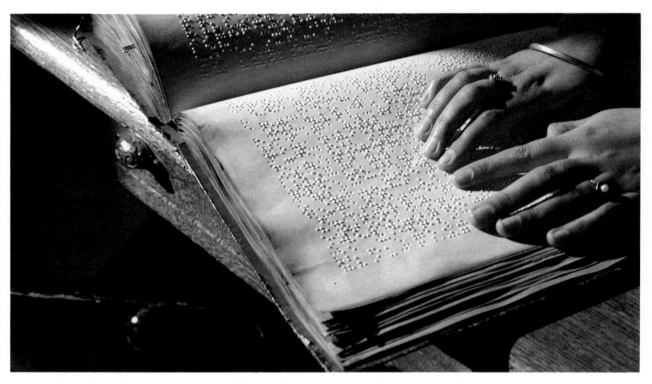

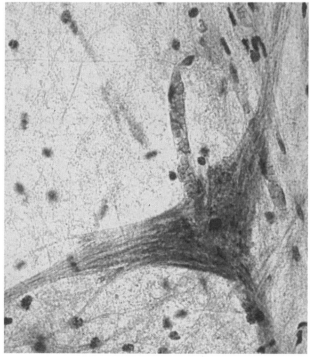

neurons emerge from the spinal cord and form an immediate synapse with a second nerve cell in a special junction-box or "vertebral ganglion" which travels all the way to the particular organ with which it is associated. Paired vertebral ganglia nestle beneath every vertebra from the base of the neck (first thoracic vertebra) to the lower back (fourth lumbar vertebra). Parasympathetic nerves emerge from the base of the brain and do not make a synapse until they reach their target organ.

Most organs receive both sympathetic and parasympathetic stimulation. These stimulations act together generally as a form of regulation – of the heartbeat, for example – for the two types of nerves tend to have independently opposing effects. It is now known that parasympathetic nerves achieve their effect by the secretion of substances related to acetylcholine – the normal neurotransmitter in vertebrate voluntary motor nerves – whereas sympathetic nerves release substances similar to the hormone epinephrine (or adrenaline). This has given rise to the terms "cholinergic" and "adrenergic" to describe the

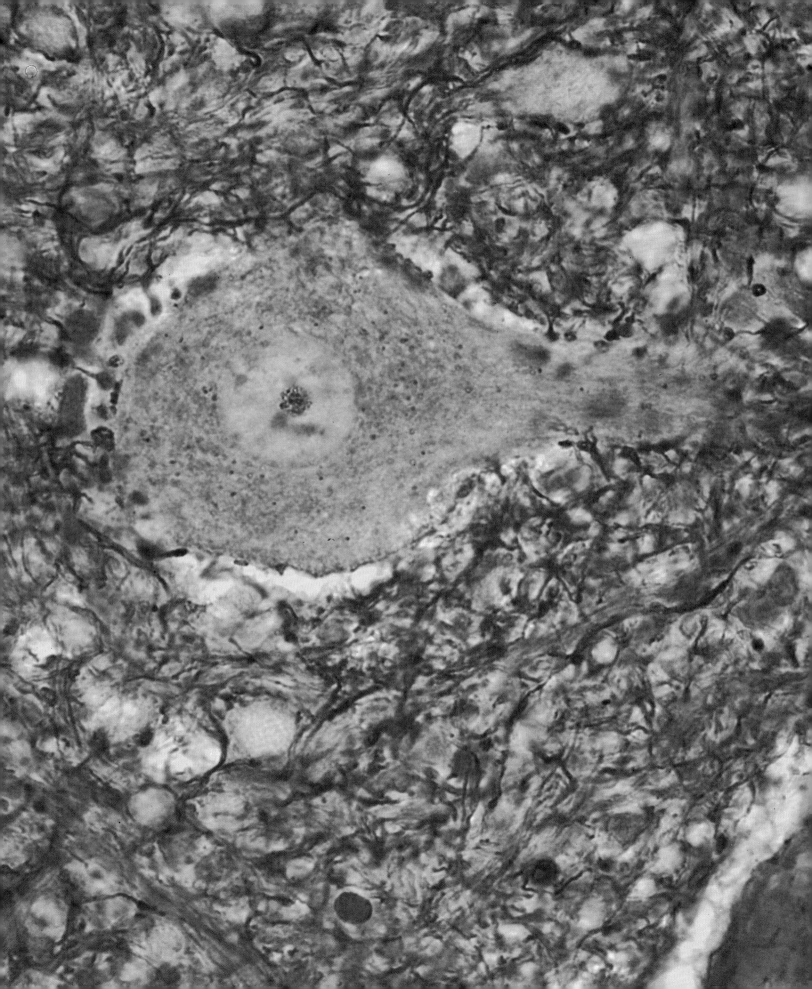

*Panting and sweating, cyclists race
to the finish. If motivation was high –
while outrunning an avalanche,
for example – the sympathetic
nervous system would assist by
regulating various body responses.*

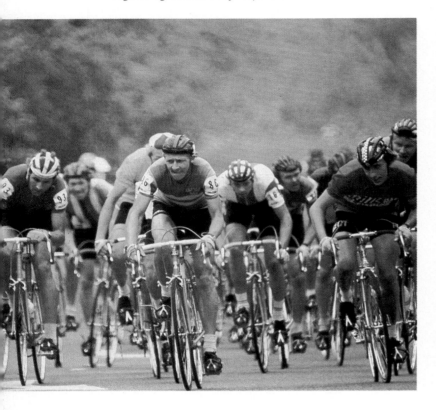

function of nerves. It is the posterior part of the pituitary body, or master gland, which lies at the base of the brain and is itself made from nervous tissue, which acts as a storehouse for the products of specialized secretory nerve cells, releasing these chemicals when called upon to do so by the autonomic system.

It is outdated to regard the nervous system as merely a communication system. Because it also relies on secretions it closely resembles the endocrine or hormonal system of the body.

Why Do Animals Have Nervous Systems?

Locomotion is an activity which requires considerable physical coordination, and as such is possible only in organisms with a system of nerves which can transmit information about the status of each part of the body to all other parts. Without a constant feedback of information about the position of your own body, for example, you would soon fall over. As you take a step the tiny compass in your inner ear informs your whole body of your state of

balance, and this is transmitted through to your feet which contract and relax many tiny toe muscles, so helping to keep you upright.

But movement brings its own problems. New situations are constantly encountered, usually by the front end, or head, of the animal; this explains why most of the sense organs, which gather information about the outside world, are positioned on the head. New situations require new responses, and a well developed nervous system is required for an individual to be able to respond in one way at one moment and in another way at the next. Nerve integration, utilizing the complex synapses, is the basis of integrated behavior.

Small animals are unable to gain very much freedom from the constraints of their immediate environments, because mobility depends upon size, and most small animals can move neither far nor fast. Large animals are highly mobile, but require a complex nervous system not just to support the mobility but also to support the large body size.

Myelin, the substance that speeds up the transmission of nerve impulses, is a characteristic of vertebrate animals, and is not found in less highly evolved invertebrate animals. This is despite the fact that some of these invertebrates are quite active and mobile, and a few are both large and active. To overcome the slowness of reaction which unmyelinated fibers impose, some large mollusks have instead evolved bundles of so-called "giant axons" which allow them to react to prey and predators every bit as fast as vertebrates.

The brain of an organism is much like the mainframe computer of a company, storing the memory of various situations and circumstances which may be recalled in the future should a similar occasion arise (although after a long period such memories may be only fragmentary).

But there is no need to resort to the brain for "first line" responses if the animal becomes, say, too hot, too cold, too dry, or is traumatized, for these circumstances can generally be adequately controlled initially by the spinal cord alone via what is known as the "reflex arc." Reflex actions are automatic, instinctive. From a stubbed toe the message travels along afferent, sensory nerve cells

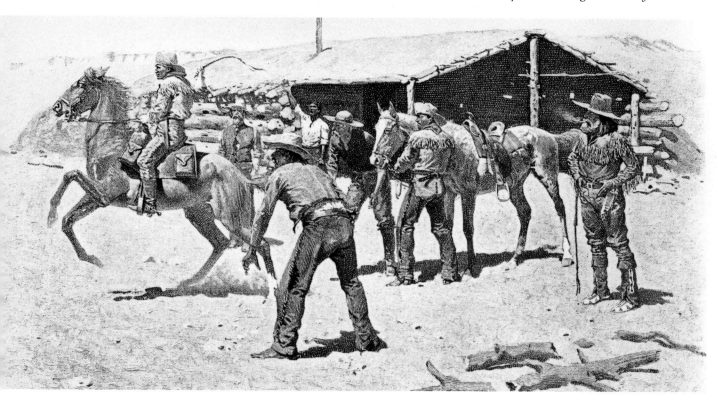

The Pony Express in order to maintain speed changed horses at towns along its route. Similarly, nerve impulses transfer their signals at synapses—and each neuron can pass on the signal to many others.

and enters the spinal cord via a lateral spinal nerve. From here signals may be sent up or down the cord depending on the severity of the pain and the amount of response required. Inside the gray matter of the spinal cord the afferent neuron synapses with an efferent motor neuron, which is stimulated and causes the toe or leg muscle to contract. The result is that in the merest fraction of a second, without any operation of the brain, the body (or part of it) has been removed from danger. Simple, primitive animals which lack a real brain live out their whole lives by little more than a series of reflex actions.

When you tread on a tack a number of additional reflex responses also occur. As you jerk your foot up, you shift your balance slightly and perhaps raise your arms to re-establish equilibrium. These reflexes are triggered by offshoots from the afferent nerve as it enters the nerve cord. The coordination of all these responses is brought about by the spinal cord. So another of the main functions of the central nervous system is to coordinate reflex activity.

Fortunately, not all normal events are as dramatic as the one just described. Every dog owner has observed that even the rattle of the dog's bowl at feeding time arouses it from a seemingly deep sleep and sends it scurrying to the kitchen. As the dog waits for its food to be prepared it salivates, so eager is it to feed. Sensory neurons from the dog's ears inform it of a familiar sound which it has come to associate with food. Motor neurons from its central nervous system as well as autonomic nerves activate the salivary glands as the dog readies itself for food. This whole activity is governed and integrated by the central nervous system, much as an integrated reflex activity. It is a similar response to that seen in reflex behavior; the central nervous system coordinates the activities of sensory and motor nerves, analyzing and processing the incoming and outgoing information.

Mention has been made of the secretory function of nerves. In a number of primitive animals which lack a true brain there are bundles of nerve cells which exist principally for their secretions. Many

Stepping onto a sharp object such as broken glass elicits the immediate response of raising the injured foot. The message (green) that instantly signals pain in the foot is sent by sensory neurons toward the brain, but is intercepted at the base of the spine, It is from there, immediately, that a message (red) is sent via the motor neurons to contract the muscles which draw back the foot. This sequence is the reflex arc.

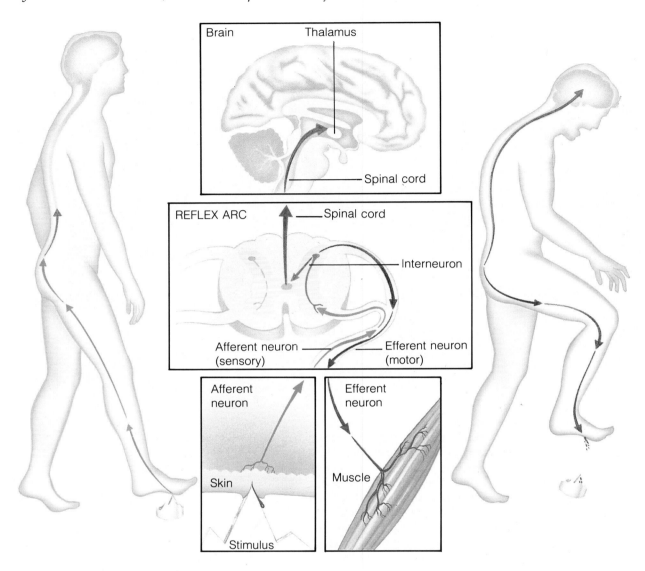

Brain

Thalamus

Spinal cord

REFLEX ARC

Spinal cord

Interneuron

Afferent neuron (sensory)

Efferent neuron (motor)

Afferent neuron

Skin

Stimulus

Efferent neuron

Muscle

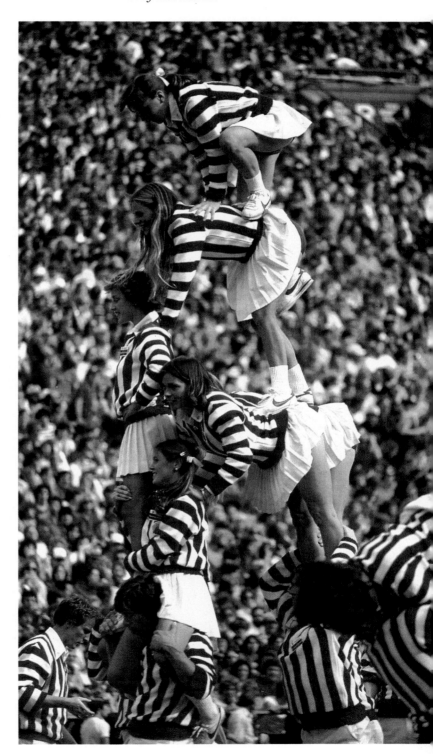

Constructing a human tower involves great muscular control and balance. At all times the body analyzes its positioning: signals pass to the cerebellum, which coordinates body movements.

crustaceans (shrimps, prawns and the like) are able to change color in order to better camouflage themselves. The color change is brought about by neurosecretory cells held in bundles just below the throat region. Such hormone function is common in this large group of animals, and recalls the neurosecretory function of the rear portion of the vertebrate's pituitary body.

Evolution is commonly thought to work on physical structures, such as leg length or tooth structure, to best suit the individual and the species to its particular environment. But as we have seen, an important function of the nervous system is to facilitate complex behavior in relation to rapidly changing circumstances. If a new food supply suddenly presents itself, species with complex nervous systems are able to exploit this new resource. As a result of new behavior specific physical modifications and adaptations to enable the species better able to avail itself of the new resource may develop.

It is well known, for example, that the Galapagos Islands off Ecuador were originally colonized by short-billed finches from the mainland. When the famous English naturalist Charles Darwin visited the islands during the last century he was struck by the many forms of bills the finches now possessed. Some were massively built for cracking open hard seeds, whereas others retained quite slender beaks for feeding on pollen and nectar. If the original immigrants had not had the behavioral capability for feeding on a range of foods – and there were no competitors on the islands – they would have continued for evermore feeding on the same sort of food that they did back home. But gradually, through many generations, their beaks became specialized for certain foods, with the result that today we can recognize 13 species of Darwin's finches. A well developed nervous system, therefore, opens up new evolutionary possibilities. On the other hand, once specialization has effectively restricted the choice of diet or environment, further evolution also is restricted.

It is important not to assume that all animals have well developed nervous systems; this is far from the case. But by considering the nervous arrangements in other creatures a better appreciation of the nervous system in humans may be reached.

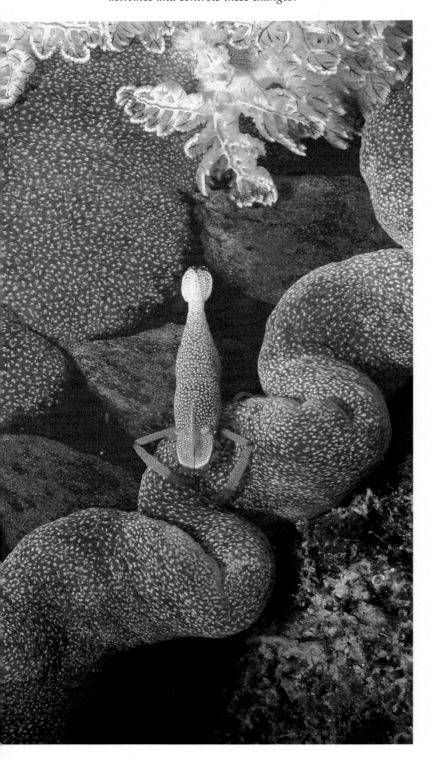

The Nervous Systems of Other Organisms

The most primitive animals, such as amebas, consist of just a single cell. All of life's vital functions are carried out within the cell membrane. By definition they have no nervous system, for a nervous system consists of a number of specialized cells. The coordination of the movements of their tiny swimming hairs (cilia) is brought about by as yet unknown mechanisms.

Sponges probably had their evolutionary origins as colonial protozoa. The article we recognize as a sponge is a sort of complex apartment house. It is not understood how the sponge cells know in which order to build their skeletons, but it is clear from anatomical study that no nervous system is involved.

The most primitive group of animals in which a nervous system is found comprises the sea anemones, jellyfish and corals. These animals have many cells in their bodies, but are organized in just two layers—an outer and an inner. (The more advanced animals have a middle layer as well.) Lying at the base of the outer layer is a so-called "nerve net" which, as its name implies, is a lattice-work of interconnecting nerve cells. Each cell gives off two or three axons which make contact with axons from other cells but do not fuse, just as in vertebrate animals a tiny synapse is left, across which the nerve impulse must jump.

Where these cells differ from those in vertebrates is that all the axons are equal—there are no dendrites—and an impulse can travel in either direction along the cell. The nerve net has a tighter mesh size around the mouth (which, in the sea anemone or coral polyp, is on the upper side at the base of the ring of tentacles) than on the column. Next time you are at the seashore take a stick, and carefully touch the mouth region of a sea anemone living in a rock pool. You will observe a fast response with the tentacles on the stimulated side arching over to investigate. Now touch the outside of the column. If you do this near the top you will get a rapid response, but if you do it near to the animal's attachment with the rock the response will be very slow indeed. Every stimulation radiates across the body through the network, and repeated stimulations travel farther than single touches.

The very first traces of nervous specialization are

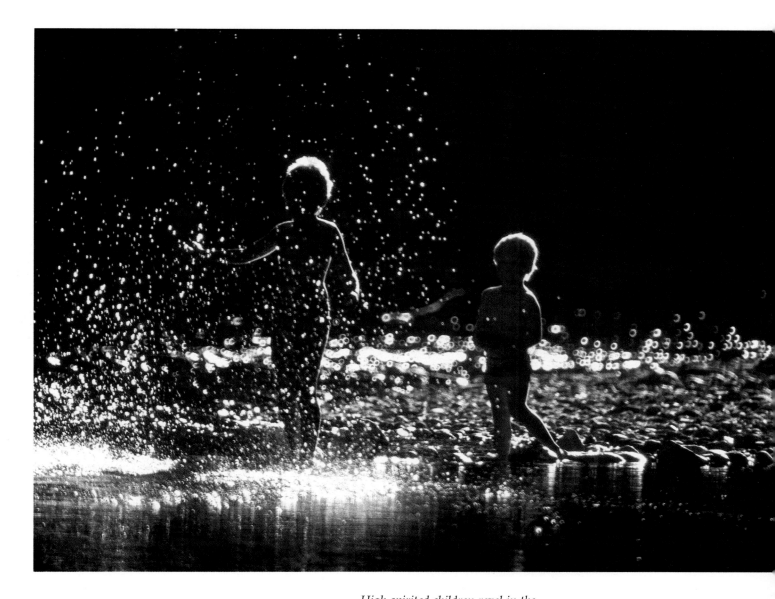

High-spirited children revel in the delight of splashing about in a fountain. All direct sensations—both pleasant and unpleasant—are the result of sensory nerve impulses being interpreted by the brain.

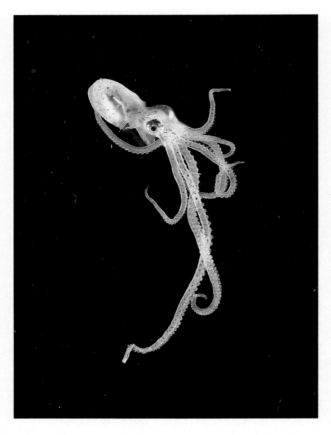

The giant unmyelinated axons of an octopus are two to three millimeters thick and pass nerve impulses at up to 75 feet per second. In humans, this speed is matched in myelinated axons a thousandth of this size.

direction can be seen in the flatworms, those little black or gray flattened, jellylike creatures found under stones, in freshwater ponds and streams. If you look at one of these animals closely, you will see a pair of crescent-shaped pale patches at one end. These are the eyes, and indicate which end is the head. They are simple structures, unable to discriminate more than the presence of light, for these vulnerable creatures shun the light.

Flatworms have a nervous system with distinct nerve tracts; they also have distinct concentrations of nerve cells near the eyes. These are called "cerebral ganglia" to underscore their brainlike function. Running rearward from the cerebral ganglia are two thick bands of nerve cells forming distinct nerve cords. This is the earliest creature in which such an arrangement is found, but it appears to have been a good design for it occurs in almost all subsequent groups.

At this point in animal evolution there arose a revolutionary new design. The bodies of animals became split up into many segments, each one containing a basic set of vital organs. The first group to show segmentation was that containing the earthworms and leeches. In these animals the segmentation is clearly visible on the outside of the body. Each segment receives a paired offshoot from a nerve cell ganglion, and the ganglia in adjacent segments are in touch with one another. As the earthworm pumps its way through the soil the ganglia are in constant contact with those immediately in front and behind it. But if the whole worm is violently stimulated, as would happen if it were attacked by a bird, the whole body is able to react instantly and effectively. This is brought about by the existence of three so-called "giant fibers" running from the frontmost segment to the rearmost, and in contact with each segmental ganglion.

Giant fibers allow a much more rapid conduction of nervous impulse than normal fibers do. The chances are that the head of the worm will encounter danger first. Here, a quite well formed cerebral ganglion, together with another ganglion lying underneath the gullet, form a workable "brain," although this is not in total command of the whole body. If an earthworm is cut in two, the rear half which is not in contact with the brain

seen in some species of sea anemone in which there are one or two clearly marked conduction paths along which impulses travel more quickly. It seems as if sea anemones are also able to discriminate between different types of environmental phenomena such as food or danger by the intensity and frequency of the stimulations.

Although there is a concentration of nerve cells at one end of the sea anemone's body, this is in no sense a brain. In all higher animals zoologists recognize the principle of cephalization, that is the development of a distinct head region. The evolutionary pressures on animals are toward increasing mobility, so that the environment may be used more completely.

Mobility, as has been explained, brings its own problems, many of which can be solved by the animal gathering and sorting environmental information from the part of the body which leads in locomotion. The first evolutionary steps in this

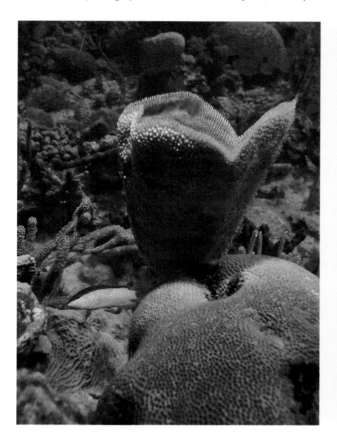 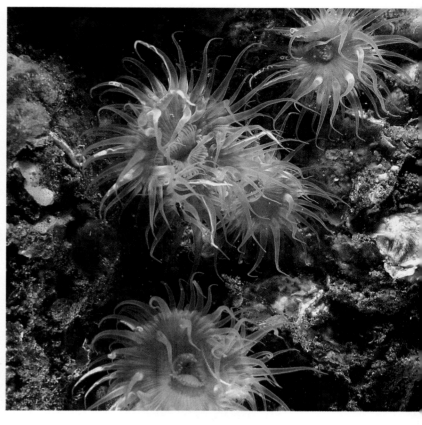

remains as alive and active as the front half. The function of the brain, then, is merely to integrate and coordinate the activities of the segmental ganglia, and the body as a whole. It is interesting to note in passing that many marine segmented worms are adapted to cast off the egg- or sperm-laden rear halves of their bodies at breeding time.

Animals with jointed limbs – principally the crustaceans, insects and spiders – have nervous systems not much more developed than those of the segmented worms. Basically, they have a cerebral ganglion lying in the head, between the eyes, and another on the side below their gut. A pair of nerves then pass rearward, with a swelling in each segment from which emerge the short nerves to control the particular activity of each segment. The function of the brain is to integrate the otherwise uncoordinated actions of the various independent segmental units. A decapitated wasp is able to walk – an activity which requires the careful integration of the movement of its six legs.

The mollusks represent a higher level of evolution, although to look at a slug or a snail one might be forgiven for doubting this. The fact is that the squids, cuttlefish and octopuses, are the most highly developed of all invertebrate creatures. Modern underwater television photography has brought the lives of these little understood creatures to mass attention. Squids and their relatives have a genuine brain, encased in a cartilaginous cranium for protection.

Characteristic of these creatures is a series of giant nerve cells running all down the body. When startled they can contract the mantle (the part of the body that forms the hood of the octopus) with such force that water forced from a narrow siphon drives them like a jet airplane. The eye of the squid is the most advanced of any non-vertebrate animal, equipped exactly like the human eye with cornea, iris, focusable lens and retina.

Within the sponge "messenger" substances are carried by ameboid cells in the sponge walls. A primitive system occurs in organisms such as jellyfish; it is diffuse and comprises a network of nerve cells in contact with each other. Flatworms are the simplest creatures in which there is a centralized nervous system having cerebral ganglia and two nerve cords. This system is further developed in earthworms, in which lateral nerves branch off the ventral nerve cord in each body segment. In present-day insects the nervous system is sufficiently complex to control flight. The nervous system is most highly developed in humans.

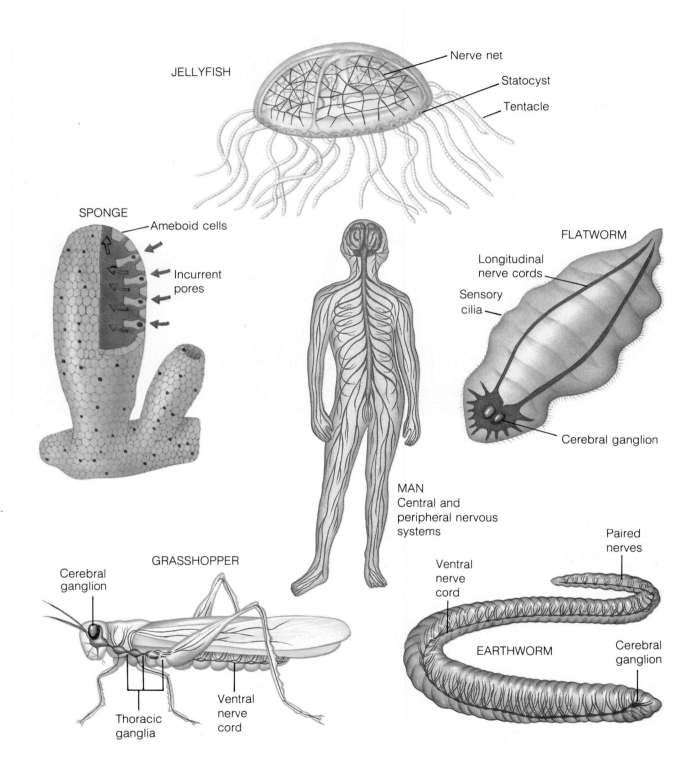

JELLYFISH

Nerve net

Statocyst

Tentacle

SPONGE

Ameboid cells

Incurrent pores

FLATWORM

Longitudinal nerve cords

Sensory cilia

Cerebral ganglion

MAN
Central and peripheral nervous systems

GRASSHOPPER

Cerebral ganglion

Thoracic ganglia

Ventral nerve cord

Ventral nerve cord

Paired nerves

EARTHWORM

Cerebral ganglion

The spines of sea urchins have an outer layer that contains sensory cells which form the major part of the animal's sensory system. In addition, the spines are used for locomotion.

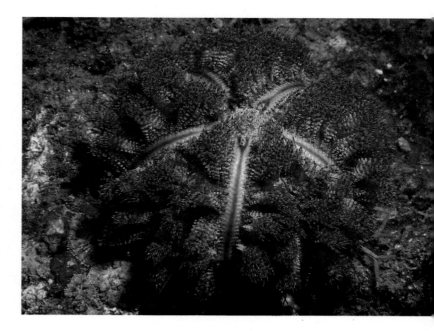

The last remaining major group of invertebrates to be considered is that to which the starfish, sea urchins and sea cucumbers belong. They all have a simple nervous system, arranged in two layers. The upper, outside, layer is mainly sensory and forms a distinct nerve ring around the mouth and a ventral nerve running along each of its five arms. The deeper layer is motor, and runs to the muscles in the arms, spines and the curious tube feet characteristic of this group of animals. Each arm is independent of all the others and there is no brain. If a starfish is damaged, and loses an arm, four new arms and a new central disk soon regrow from that single arm – a feat which no vertebrate animal can emulate.

Finally, there is an obscure little group of animals which most people would ignore on the beach. They are the group to which the sea squirts belong; spongelike encrusting animals often found in rock pools. These unprepossessing creatures occupy the middle ground between invertebrate and vertebrate animals, for their larval forms all have a stiffening rod reminiscent of, but not identical to, the vertebral column. For the first time in evolution there is a dorsal nerve cord (one which runs along the back of the animal) which is hollow. These are the characteristics of the nervous systems of all vertebrates, including humans.

In the true vertebrates all that remains visible of the segmentation clearly seen in the earthworms is the row of vertebrae which together make up the spine. Cephalization has developed, which means that a distinct head is present. The collected nerve cells from primitive segments now form the brain and the cranial nerves – some of which form the parasympathetic nervous system. The nervous systems of all vertebrates – fishes, amphibians, reptiles, birds and mammals – are built to the same plan of a brain, hollow dorsal nerve cord and "segmental" ganglia. If the brain is removed from a vertebrate death almost always follows instantly. It is characteristic that the brain is intimately involved in the body's vital functions; other nerve plexuses are incapable of supporting life without the brain.

The human nervous system, then, is certainly among the most complex in the animal kingdom, and together with the most remarkable brain of all has brought the human race to the peak of natural supremacy.

Unlike most other vital systems of the human body which are localized, the peripheral nervous system is widely spread. As the nerves travel outward from the spinal cord they send off branches which divide and subdivide so covering all parts of the body. The nerve net is denser in the sensitive parts of the body's surface, such as the fingertips and lips, than on the less sensitive regions, such as the back. Sensory nerves end in touch, temperature or chemical receptors, depending upon location. Some regions, such as the tongue, are well endowed with all three.

The nerves which make up the peripheral nervous system come mainly from the spinal cord. Aggregations of nerves, called ganglia, just outside the spinal cord help to sift the information flow and integrate whatever other actions are needed. Few nerves actually emerge from the brain and travel around the body. Some to the face, teeth and mouth do, but below the head the only major cranial nerve is the vagus, or the parasympathetic part of the autonomic nervous system. All bodily movements are controlled by spinal nerves; this is why paralysis follows from serious back injury, and from the point of injury downward. It is through the nerves that we experience the events of everyday life – all the sensations encountered by the senses, of course, but also everything we learn or remember. The nervous system is more than just a network within the body – it is more like the plumbing, electrics and interior decoration in a large modern building.

41

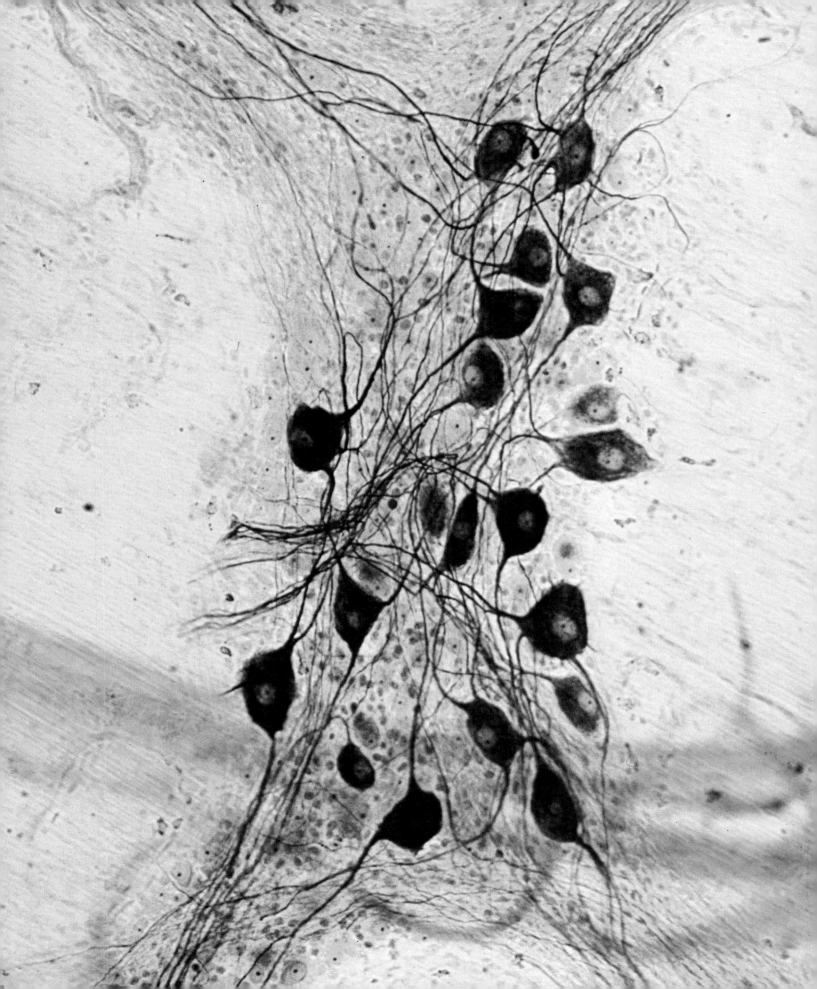

Chapter 3

Ionic Impulses

Most nerve cells, or neurons, resemble a tall bushy-topped tree in miniature. They have a single axon (the narrow part of the nerve cell) and many dendrites (the spiky parts). Dendrites are fairly short projections about one-twentyfifth of an inch long, and they branch repeatedly to form a treelike mass of branches, the dendrite tree. The tips of dendrites carry hundreds of much smaller projections, the dendritic spines, with a total of 40,000 and 100,000 spines on every cell. They are the receiving areas for information that arrives from other nerve cells. Each neuron can therefore receive messages from many hundreds of other nerve cells. These messages are integrated within the cell body, and any resulting nerve impulse is carried from the cell to the next in line in the chain along the axon.

The axon is the longest projection from the neuron. It generally emerges from the cell body at a raised region, the axon hillock. An axon may be only one-hundredth of an inch or so in length, or may stretch three feet or more in a nerve that links the brain with the lower abdomen. The width or diameter of an axon varies from about one-tenthousandth of an inch up to about one thousandth of an inch in humans and other mammals, but in invertebrates axon diameters are often much larger. The squid, for example, has some giant axons with diameters of around one-twelfth of an inch.

The axon rarely branches along its length and where it does so the branches, or collaterals, generally run off at right angles to the main axon. The end of the axon does branch, but never so profusely as dendrites. Axon branches may make contact with dendrites, the cell body or the axon of other nerve cells, or they may end at muscle fibers. Each axon branch usually ends in a knoblike swelling, the terminal bouton or button, and it is these swellings that are involved in making connections with other nerves or muscles.

Nerve impulses shoot along fibers, in times measured in milliseconds, enabling fast reactions to their messages. Shown here is part of the vagus nerve in the intestines, where it delivers messages from the brain that activate smooth muscles in the gut and stimulate the secretion of digestive juices. The nuclei of individual nerve cells show up as dark patches, interconnected by branching dendrites.

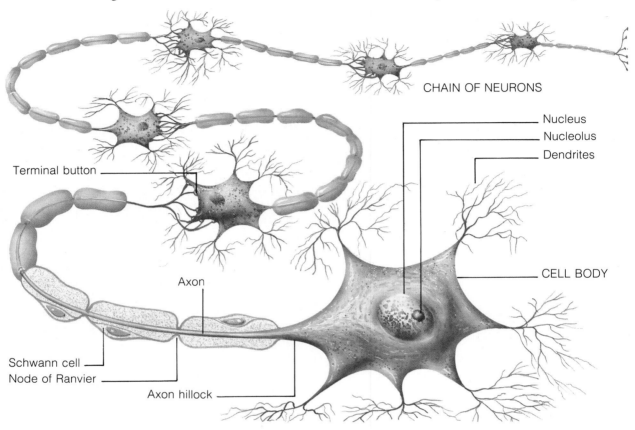

Neurons (below) comprise a cell body with dendrites and an axon with a branched tip, from which messages pass to the next neuron. Organelles carry chemicals along the axon like boxcars along track.

A tree with spreading branches closely resembles a nerve cell with its branching processes. The similarity led to these nerve structures being called dendrites, from dendron, *the Greek for tree.*

CHAIN OF NEURONS

Nucleus

Nucleolus

Dendrites

Terminal button

CELL BODY

Axon

Schwann cell

Node of Ranvier

Axon hillock

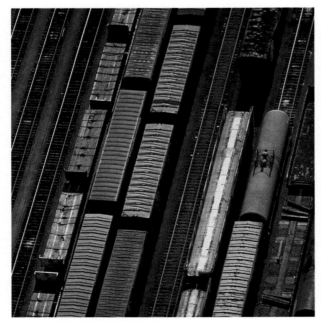

In terms of ultrastructure, a nerve cell is similar to most other cells in the body. It is surrounded by a membrane, the plasma membrane. The membrane contains protein molecules and lipids (fatty molecules), and has a major role in the electrical activity of the neuron.

Within the membrane lies the cytoplasm, a soup of chemicals which includes large proteins and small salts such as sodium and potassium chloride. There are also the usual cell organelles, which control the various functions of the cell. Each nerve cell characteristically contains near its nucleus a dense aggregation of rough endoplasmic reticulum known as the Nissl substance, which probably manufactures the specific membrane proteins that are used by nerve cells. Transmission of electrical signals along a nerve axon requires energy, and this is provided by the mitochondria. In this way, the cell body provides all the essential materials for the whole cell to function properly. If it is separated

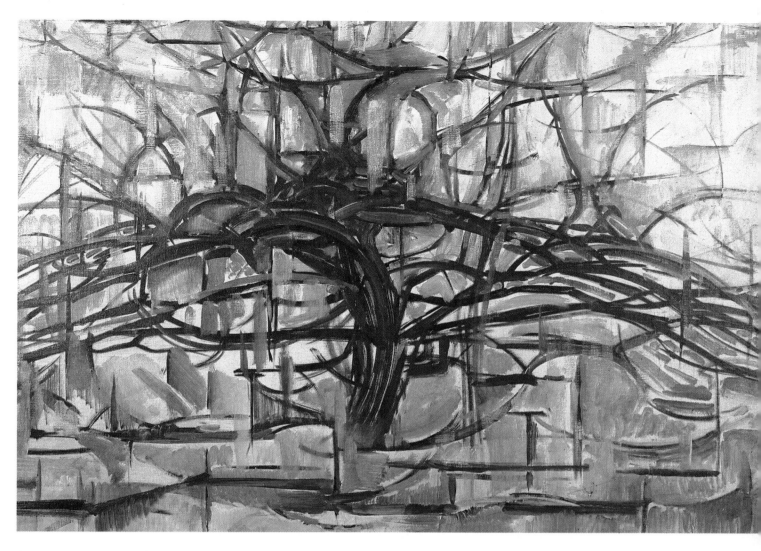

from its nucleus, as for example when a nerve is cut, the axon dies.

Nerve cells also contain minute tubes and fibers. Microtubules are hollow tubular structures which act as a sort of skeleton to maintain the shape of the cell. Neurotubules or neurofilaments, found only in nerve cells, are even finer. Also tubular in shape, they are particularly common in long axons. Both types of filaments seem to be involved in transporting material like a sort of conveyor belt between the cell body and the nerve terminals, a process known as axonal transport. Their "cargoes" are probably chemicals involved in the transmission of signals from cell to cell.

Natural Nerve Glue

The early anatomists found components which they believed held or "glued" the nerve cells together. Later studies using microscopes showed that this neuroglia (literally, nerve glue) is com-posed of separate cells that are so numerous they often outnumber nerve cells by ten to one. The glial cells support the neurons and give the nervous system its structural framework. They also form a barrier between the bloodstream and the nervous tissue, letting through only certain essential substances such as oxygen, water and some sugars.

There are several different types of glial cell in the central nervous system. The most common are oligodendrocytes, which contain many microtubules and have a special function in providing protective sheaths around the long axons that connect various parts of the system.

The peripheral nervous system has a single type of glial cell called Schwann cell, for their discoverer Theodor Schwann. In the simplest arrangement, involving small axons, one or a group of axons are embedded in a single Schwann cell. Those around the larger axons form a complex structure. As a nerve cell and its axon begin to develop, the

Theodor Schwann

Champion of Cell Theory

Applying his brilliant mind to physiology, Theodor Schwann made important discoveries in digestion and fermentation, established "cell theory" and identified the so-called "Schwann cells". Most of his achievements were packed into the first years of his career, his later life being devoted to religion and inventing machinery.

He was born on December 7, 1810 in the town of Neuss, now in West Germany. According to all reports he was something of a model student and a brilliant all-rounder, dedicated to his work. After abandoning his career in the Church, he studied medicine at the Universities of Bonn, Würzburg and Berlin, and was lucky enough to obtain a position as assistant to the eminent German physiologist Johannes Müller at the Museum of Anatomy in Berlin.

Initially he concerned himself with the processes of digestion. He successfully isolated the chemical responsible for protein digestion from the stomach lining and called it pepsin from the Greek word meaning "to digest". This enzyme — as it is now classified — was the first isolated from animal tissues.

One of his discoveries that did not find favor among

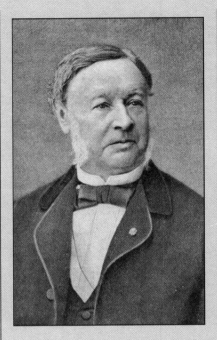

contemporary scientists was his belief that the fermentation of sugar was the result of a life process — that is, yeast was made up of living organisms. It was the work of Louis Pasteur a generation later that finally proved his observations correct.

Schwann is perhaps best known, however, for his cell theory. He maintained that all animals and plants consist entirely of cells or products of cells, and that the life of these cells is subordinate to the life of the whole organism. His closest friend Matthias Schleiden had put forward a similar theory relating to plants

but it was Schwann who effectively applied the theory to both animals and plants.

He defined the cell as "a layer around a nucleus" and correctly identified an egg as a single cell which develops into a highly complex organism.

He outlined his theories in *Microscopical Researches on the Similarity in the Structure of Growth of Animals and Plants*. The preface to the English edition deemed "the discoveries which it unfolds as worthy to be ranked among the most important steps by which the science of physiology has ever been advanced."

In his investigations into the different types and arrangements of cells, he identified what are now known as Schwann cells. These cells make up the myelin sheaths which surround the peripheral axons. Each cell wraps many layers of its plasma membrane around a single axon.

In 1847 Schwann was appointed Professor of Anatomy at Liège University. He turned his attentions to religion once again and lost something of the passion which he had applied to his earlier medical studies. He took up inventing, specializing in machinery for the mining industry. He died while visiting Cologne in 1882.

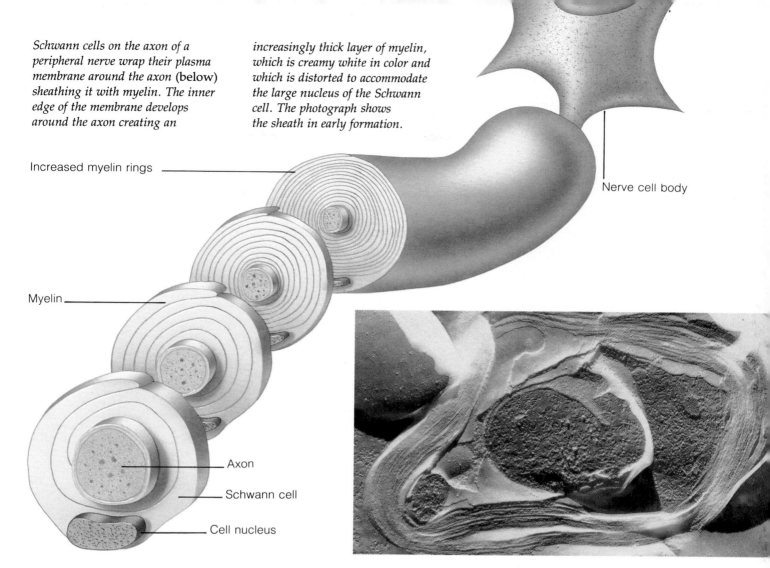

Schwann cells on the axon of a peripheral nerve wrap their plasma membrane around the axon (below) sheathing it with myelin. The inner edge of the membrane develops around the axon creating an

increasingly thick layer of myelin, which is creamy white in color and which is distorted to accommodate the large nucleus of the Schwann cell. The photograph shows the sheath in early formation.

Nerve cell body

Increased myelin rings

Myelin

Axon

Schwann cell

Cell nucleus

Schwann cell wraps itself round and round the axon up to 80 times, forming a double spiral round it. Each layer of membrane has a fatty layer, and the result is that the Schwann cell binding forms a tight, thick fatty sheath around the axon which insulates it from its neighbors. The sheath is myelin, and myelinated axons occur only in vertebrate animals.

Where an axon arises from the axon hillock it remains naked for a short distance, called the initial segment, before becoming surrounded by myelin. The sheath is not continuous, however. Each Schwann cell is between one-seventyfifth and three-fiftieths of an inch long and is separated from the next by a small gap. The gaps are known as nodes of Ranvier for the French pathologist who first described them in 1871. The myelin sheath therefore has many minute gaps along its length where the axon is exposed to the surrounding tissues and its fluids. An axon branches only at a node.

Each axon with its glial sheath constitutes a nerve fiber, and what is usually regarded as a single nerve is actually made up of thousands of such fibers, in a way much resembling a telephone cable. These nerve trunks contain a mixture of axons of large and small diameters, of myelinated and unmyelinated axons, and of axons carrying sensory information to the central nervous system. They also contain motor axons carrying commands to the muscles and glands. The various fibers can be distinguished only by their diameters and the presence or absence of myelin; the axons of sensory and motor fibers are identical and so cannot be distinguished visually in a nerve trunk.

In both the peripheral and central nervous systems, the presence of myelin sheaths gives the nerves a white appearance, whereas unmyelinated ones appear gray. For this reason the central areas of the cerebral cortex (in the brain) and of the spinal cord, composed mainly of unmyelinated cells, are

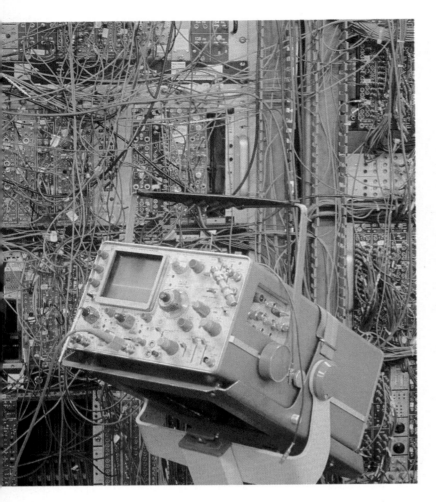

An oscilloscope, here being used to measure voltages in a complex electronic circuit, is also employed by researchers studying changes in potential across axon membranes as an impulse travels along a nerve.

gray and consequently called gray matter. The outer areas — which consist of the myelinated fibers running from these cell bodies — form the white matter.

Electrical Signals and Nerves

Animals have been using electricity for many millions of years. The voltages, unlike those used in industry and in the home, are very small, of the order of a few thousandths of a volt (a few millivolts). In nerves and muscles the electric current — which constitutes the nerve impulse — is carried by charged particles called ions. Molecules of common salt (sodium chloride), for example, are each made up of an atom of sodium and one of chlorine. When sodium chloride is dissolved in water, as it is in the body, sodium atoms become positively charged ions and chlorine atoms become negatively charged ions. The movement of such ions through a solution constitutes the electric current.

The passage of a nerve impulse is accompanied by a peak in electrical voltage called an action potential. Its passage depends on the fact that, in all nerve cells, there is a potential difference across the membrane between the outside and the inside. When the nerve is at rest, the inside is electrically negative to the outside.

To record this potential, even with giant squid axons, scientists use microelectrodes. These are usually made from fine glass capillary tubes, or micropipettes, in which the diameter of the tip can be smaller than one-twentyfivethousandth of an inch. The micropipettes are filled with a strong salt solution, usually potassium chloride, which conducts electrical activity from the nerve to a fine wire in the wider end of the micropipette. Because the electrical signals are very small, they are amplified and then recorded on an oscilloscope.

The Resting Nerve

To record the potential across the membrane in a resting nerve the tip of a microelectrode, called the active electrode, is gently pushed through the membrane into the cell body or axon. A reference electrode is placed outside the cell in the surrounding fluid or tissue, and the difference in potential between the two electrodes recorded by the oscilloscope. This is called the resting potential of the nerve. All excitable cells — nerves, muscles and sensory cells — have a resting potential.

It has been known since the end of the last century that the cytoplasm of axons contains more potassium ions and fewer sodium ions than the blood or fluid outside cells. The concentration of potassium is 20 to 100 times higher inside a nerve than outside, while the sodium concentration is 5 to 15 times higher outside than in. In 1902 the German physiologist Julius Bernstein suggested that this unequal distribution was responsible for producing the resting potential. With a few modifications his ideas still form the basis of modern ionic theory of resting potential.

Moving Molecules

Molecules in solution move continually from areas of high concentration to ones of low concentration; they move down concentration gradients. Thus a spoonful of sugar in the bottom of a cup of coffee, if left long enough, dissolves to sweeten the whole cup evenly. Ions in solution are electrically

A fireboat (below) pumps up water from the river in which it floats, to extinguish a fire. A similar pumping mechanism is thought to occur in an axon in the sodium-potassium pump (bottom). At resting stage an axon contains more potassium ions than sodium ions, whereas outside the cell there are more sodium than potassium ions. As a nerve impulse approaches, the potassium ions are "pumped" out and sodium ions enter the cell, increasing its positive charge. When the impulse arrives the electric potential peaks. The impulse passes and the sodium ions are "pumped" out; the potassium returns, restoring the resting potential.

charged, and tend to move down comparable electrical gradients. A mixed solution of potassium and sodium chloride can be separated using a membrane having tiny holes or pores in it such that the potassium and chloride ions can move freely through the pores but the sodium ions cannot. The membrane of a nerve cell is rather like this, being much less permeable to sodium than it is to potassium and chloride.

The nerve cell membrane can therefore be pictured as containing many pores, often called channels, through which ions can move. Because there is more potassium inside the cell than outside, there is a natural tendency for potassium ions to move out of the cell down their concentration gradient. But as they do, they carry positive charges out of the cell, making the inside more negative. This causes a potential to be built up across the membrane.

As the negative charges accumulate inside the cell they tend to attract back the positively charged potassium ions. Eventually the effect of this potential just cancels out the effect of the concentration gradient and the numbers of ions

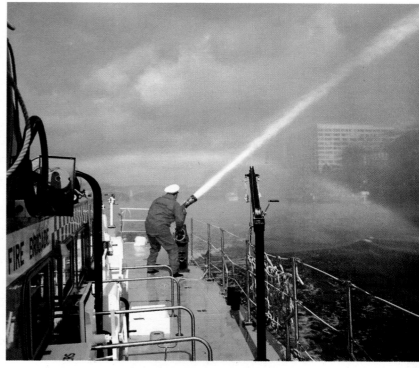

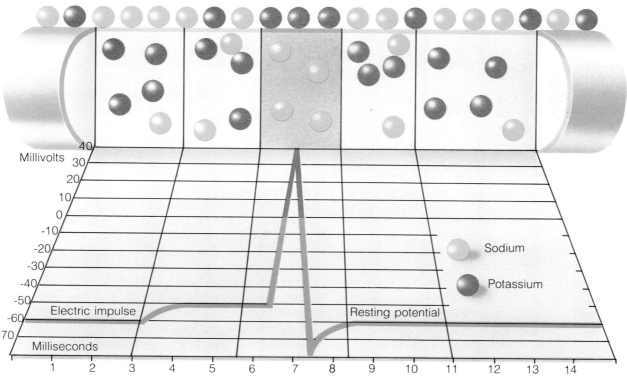

Protein gates in an axon membrane sense the approach of a nerve impulse and change shape to allow sodium ions in. After all the gates have been opened they automatically close, and sodium is forced out again.

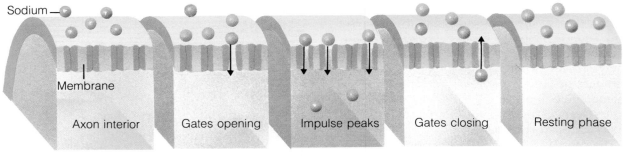

Sodium

Membrane

Axon interior   Gates opening   Impulse peaks   Gates closing   Resting phase

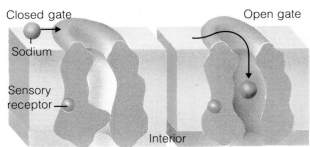

Closed gate   Open gate

Sodium

Sensory receptor

Interior

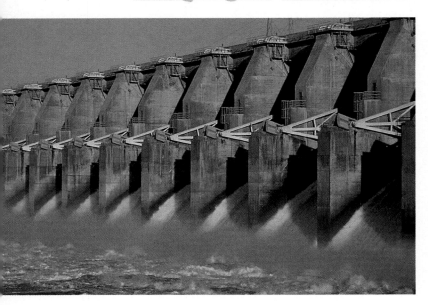

Dam gates can be operated to hold water back or to let it through to the river below. The number of gates open can vary to control the flow of water. In the same way sodium gates in an axon membrane bar the entry of sodium ions into the axon or permit it.

entering and leaving the cell are the same (there is no net movement of ions). The potential at which this occurs is the equilibrium potential for potassium, and its value depends on the various ionic concentrations.

In 1962 researchers succeeded in changing the ion concentration inside an axon. They made a small rubber roller, like a miniature lawn roller, and used it to squeeze the cytoplasm out of an isolated squid axon. They then replaced it with solutions of various concentrations by means of a micropipette inserted into the cut end of the nerve. As expected, when the internal potassium was increased, so was the resting potential; when it was reduced the resting potential decreased and became zero, when the internal concentration equalled that outside. So it seems that the unequal distribution of potassium could indeed be largely responsible for the resting potential which, as has been seen, is nearly — but not quite — equal to the potassium equilibrium potential.

It remains to consider the sodium and chloride ions. In fact, although chloride ions do move in and out of the cell, they have been found to have little effect on the resting potential and so need not be considered further. But what about the effects of sodium? Its concentration outside the nerve is higher than inside, and because the cell membrane is not totally impervious to sodium, sodium tends to move down its concentration gradient into the cell. In addition, the positively charged sodium ions will be attracted toward the internal negativity. But the low permeability of the membrane to sodium permits it to enter only slowly, making the inside of the cell slightly less negative. For this reason, the membrane potential is less than the value calculated by potassium concentration.

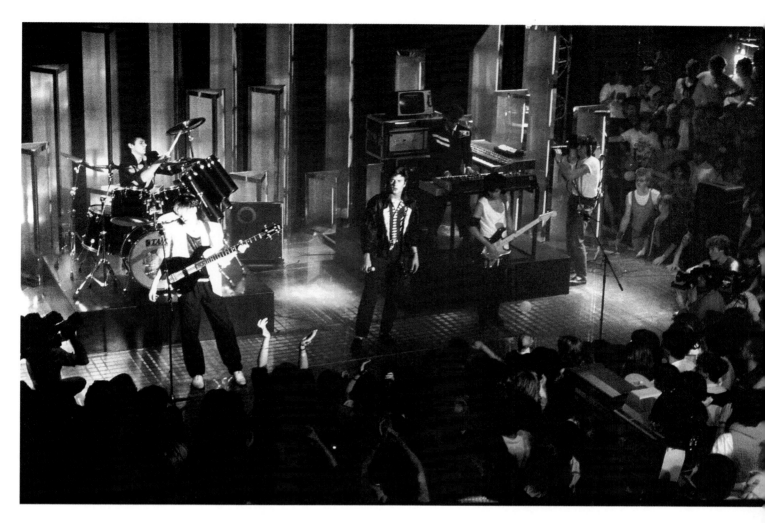

Sodium must also be removed from the cell, or its continued accumulation inside would gradually neutralize the internal negativity and the resting potential would drop to zero. This removal demands energy. Just as with potassium, the expulsion of sodium appears to be driven by an active pump. The movements of both are known to be linked, and the mechanism involved is called the coupled sodium-potassium pump.

The Nerve Impulse

A nerve impulse is a tiny burst of electric current, accompanied by a sudden voltage change. Research has shown how this voltage is generated. During the passage of a nerve impulse, the cell becomes depolarized and there is a brief but marked change in membrane potential. The effect lasts about one-thousandth of a second (one millisecond) before the inside of the nerve cell again becomes negative. At first it becomes more negative than the resting potential, before the resting potential is re-established.

The amplified sound at a pop concert is registered in the brain by a greater number of impulses than if the sound were softer. The rate of generation of impulses in the ear depends on a sound's loudness.

Alan Hodgkin and Andrew Huxley

Giant Squids and the Sodium Pump

In 1963 Alan Hodgkin and Andrew Huxley were awarded the Nobel Prize in Physiology and Medicine. This honor was bestowed on them in recognition of their pioneering work into the movements of ions in the excitement of the nerve membranes. Their contribution to the understanding of nerve impulse transmission is of great importance and their methods are used today by many scientists in this field.

Hodgkin was born on February 15, 1914 in Banbury, England and educated at Trinity College, Cambridge. After working briefly at the Rockefeller Institute, he moved to the Woods Hole Marine Biological Laboratories in Massachusetts. Here he was able to begin research into the nerve fibers of squids—these animals, and crabs, were to be the main source of Hodgkin's information because they have relatively large nerve fibers.

Huxley was born on November 22, 1917 in London and was the grandson of Darwin's distinguished friend Thomas Huxley. He too graduated from Trinity College, Cambridge, gaining an MA in 1941.

The research of both men was cut short by World War II and while Hodgkin worked on

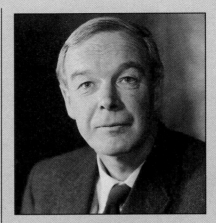

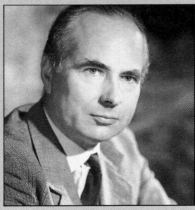

radar for the Air Ministry in England, Huxley carried out research for Anti-aircraft Command. After the war, both men joined forces at Cambridge in a partnership that was to be very influential in the field of physiology.

At the beginning of the twentieth century J. Bernstein had put forward a theory concerning the bioelectric currents of the nervous system.

He believed a "resting" potential was the result of the permeability of the nerve membrane to potassium ions. Hodgkin and Huxley set about measuring electrochemical behavior in the the axons of the giant squid.

They placed a microelectrode and a capillary tube filled with seawater into the axon to monitor the ions in and around the cell. In this way they were able to record electrical changes across the cell. It was shown that at first the inside of the cell was negative (the resting potential) and the outside positive, but that during the peak of the nerve impulse, the conditions were reversed.

Hodgkin and Huxley worked out a theory to account for their findings—the "sodium pump" theory as it has become known. They showed that potassium ions are plentiful inside a nerve cell whereas the exterior is rich in sodium ions. When a nerve impulse is transmitted, however, sodium ions flood into the cell pushing potassium ions out. The chemicals return to their natural distribution once the impulse has passed, ready for the next transmission.

Hodgkin outlined their findings in his book *Conduction of the Nervous Impulse*, which was published in 1963.

In a nerve, then, an action potential is produced when the cell is depolarized beyond a certain minimum threshold value. The potential is constant for a given axon, generally between +30 and +50 mV. Increasing the initial depolarization beyond the threshold value does not increase the action potential, which is therefore said to be "all or none." So, because the size of the action potential cannot be varied, the only way information carried by an axon can be varied is to increase or decrease the rate at which impulses are produced. In axons from the sense organs, for example, the rate of impulse production is related to the strength of the stimulus — the louder a sound, for example, the greater is the number of impulses per second sent from the ear to the brain.

The ionic basis of action potentials was worked out mainly by Cole and Curtis in the United States and by Alan Hodgkin and Andrew Huxley and their colleagues in England. In 1939 both groups demonstrated that, during the passage of a nerve impulse, the membrane potential did not just fall to zero, but that there was an "overshoot" to a positive value. Ten years later Hodgkin and Katz showed that the size of the overshoot reduced when the sodium concentration outside the nerve cell dropped. It seems that the rapid change in potential from negative to positive and back is caused by a transient increase in the permeability of the plasma membrane to sodium.

To test this idea, a method of holding the membrane potential constant — now known as the voltage-clamp technique — was devised by Cole in 1949. It is used to depolarize the membrane to a known level and then hold it steady. No action potentials are produced even though the depolarization may be above the threshold of the axon, but the permeability changes and ion movements still occur and can be studied independently of potential changes.

Depolarization seems to produce an opening of sodium channels. As sodium enters the axon, it depolarizes the membrane further and so increases the permeability. The entry of positive charges makes the inside positive, and the membrane potential approaches the theoretical equilibrium. At the same time the concentration and electrical gradients decrease, the permeability soon de-

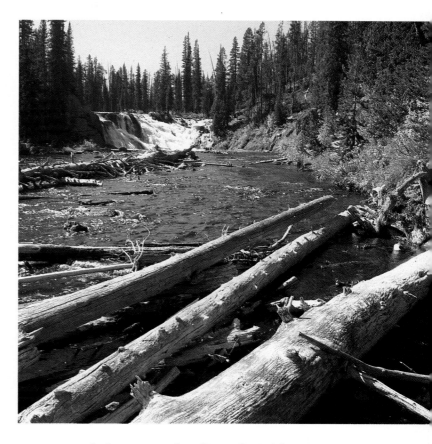

creases, and the entry of sodium diminishes in consequence.

Meanwhile the membrane's permeability to potassium ions increases until the movement of potassium out of the cell exceeds that of sodium in, so the membrane potential again becomes negative inside — the membrane repolarizes. The repolarization goes beyond the resting level, however, before the outflow of potassium ceases. The sodium-potassium pump then restores the internal and external sodium and potassium concentrations to their resting levels.

Once the increased permeability to sodium has been activated, it cannot be reactivated again for a millisecond or so. For this reason, a nerve cannot propagate a second impulse within one or two milliseconds. The normal limit to nerve transmission is therefore about 500 pulses per second (although rarely it can rise to perhaps as high as 1,000 per second).

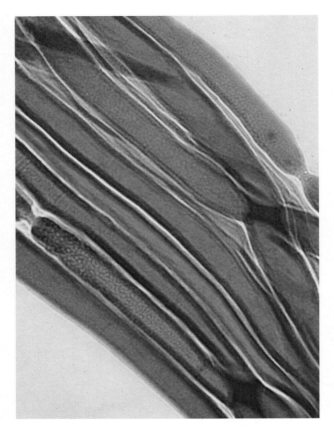

Channels, Gates and Pumps

The basis of the permeability of the membrane is the existence of channels in it that let through certain ions and not others. The channels therefore act as selective filters, and many scientists believe that they are pores in the membrane associated with particular membrane proteins. Because the permeability to both sodium and potassium can change, it is thought that each channel has molecular "gates" that can open and close to activate or inactivate the channel. The action of these gates depends on the membrane potential, and they are therefore said to be voltage-sensitive. Hodgkin and Huxley suggested in 1952 that the gates of the sodium channel might be associated with electric charges which would cause minute currents if they moved to open or close the gates. Such currents were detected in the early 1970s and are called gating currents. More recently it has become possible to place a very fine micropipette

against a small patch of membrane and so study the action of a single channel. In 1984 the molecular structure of the sodium channel was worked out by a team of Japanese researchers. It was found to consist of a single protein which spans the membrane. This protein contains four positively-charged segments which could be involved in the gating mechanism.

The sodium-potassium pump also involves a membrane protein which acts as a carrier for these ions. The protein probably combines with sodium inside the cell to form a complex molecule which moves the sodium across the cell membrane to the outside, where it is released and potassium taken up. The potassium is then transported to the inside of the membrane. The process requires energy, and the carrier molecule itself is an enzyme that splits ATP (adenosine triphosphate) to release the necessary energy.

Propagation of Action Potentials

During the action potential positive current, carried by sodium ions, enters the cell. As has been explained charges tend to move down their electrical gradient and so move down the length of the axon away from the point of entry. The charges also tend to cross the membrane to complete the electrical circuit of current flow. The current therefore tends to spread away from its point of entry and decreases in strength as it does so. This is called electrotonic conduction. The distance that the current spreads down the axon depends on the resistance offered by the cytoplasm and that offered by the membrane. The higher the membrane resistance and the lower the cytoplasm resistance, the farther the current spreads. This spread of positive current within the axon causes regions near its point of entry to become depolarized, and if the extent of depolarization reaches threshold levels an impulse is generated.

The process continues along the axon at a rate that depends on its diameter and its degree of myelination. The larger the diameter, the less the internal resistance and so the faster is the propagation of the initial depolarization and subsequent action potential. Such continuous propagation is found in unmyelinated axons which, in invertebrates, are the ones with the

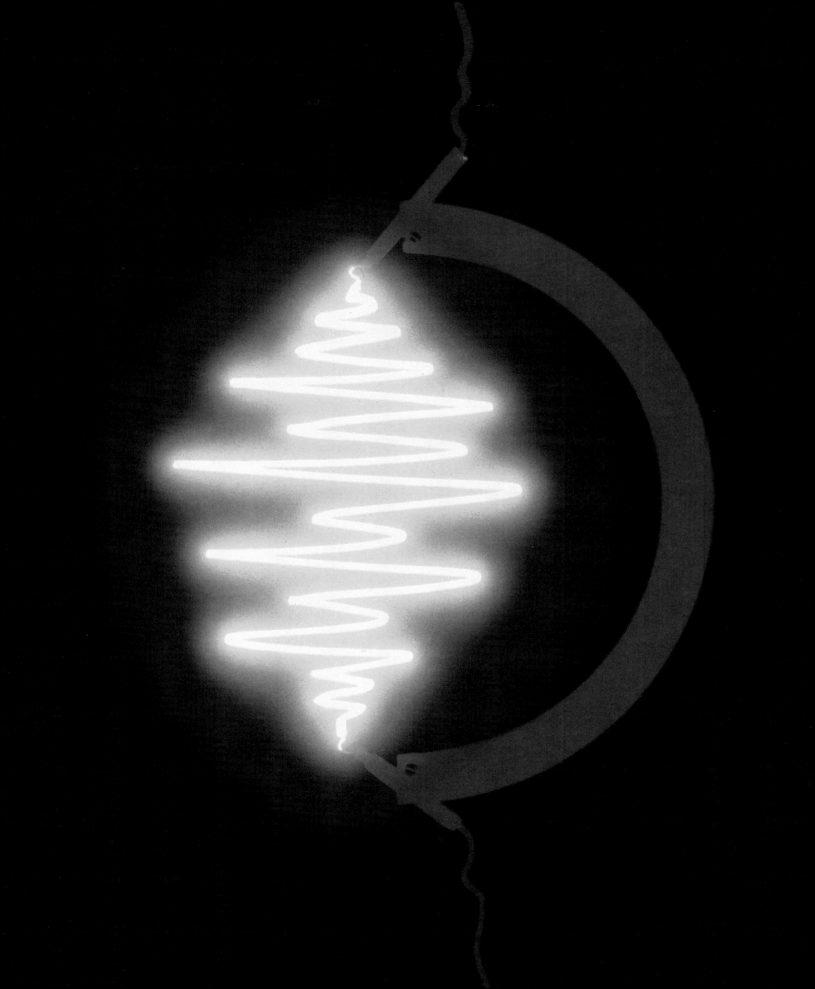

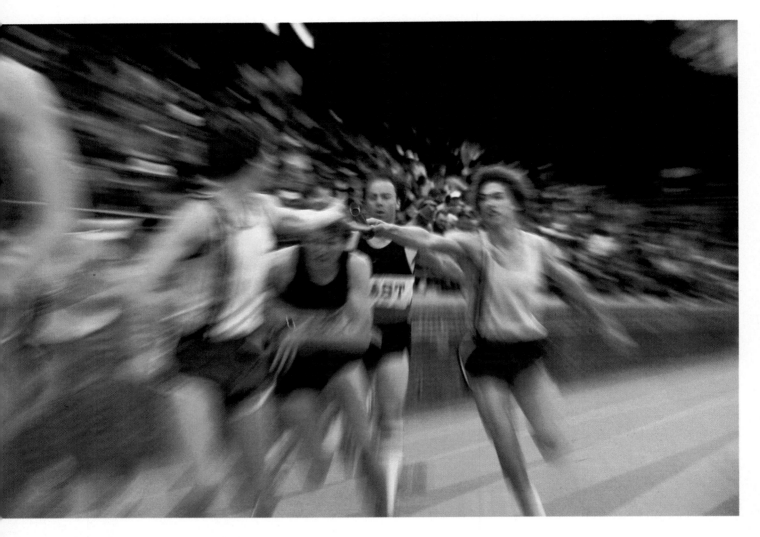

The activity at a synapse between nerve cells is like a relay race — the signal travels down the axon to the boutons, much as the baton is carried along the track by one runner, and passes across the synapse to the next nerve cell, just as the baton is handed over to the next runner.

Chemical transmitters jump across a synapse like sparks fly from a cable (below). In a motor end plate, shown attached to a striated muscle (bottom), the arrival of an impulse causes the release of the transmitter

acetylcholine, which passes the information to the muscle. The enzyme acetylcholinesterase breaks down the acetylcholine and inactivates it, resetting the mechanism before the next impulse arrives.

smallest diameters. Their rate of impulse propagation is about 8 to 24 inches per second.

The myelinated fibers' sheath of myelin is interrupted at the nodes of Ranvier and increases the resistance of the membrane to current flow. The current therefore jumps from one node to the next ("saltatory conduction") before it crosses the membrane. There are many more sodium channels at the nodes than in the membrane between them, and this results in the very fast propagation of the impulse at rates of up to 370 feet per second.

Fibers of different diameter and degrees of myelination therefore carry impulses at different speeds, and they are used for different functions in the body. The largest myelinated fibers with fast conduction velocities are used to carry sensory information to the central nervous system and to send motor commands to the muscles used in posture and movement. The unmyelinated and the smaller myelinated fibers often are present in the automatic nervous system and serve the visceral organs and blood vessels.

Nerve-to-Nerve Communication

The area where nerve transmits information to other nerves or to effectors such as muscles is known as a synapse. In most cases this involves chemical transmission between adjacent nerve cells. A typical synapse consists of a presynaptic region (for example the terminal boutons of the axon branches), the gap or synaptic cleft, and the postsynaptic region (for example the dendritic spines). The presynaptic region is often swollen to form the presynaptic knob, which contains many dense vesicles. At some synapses there is evidence that more than one transmitter chemical is bound to or associated with these vesicles. The synaptic cleft is very narrow and filled with a gluelike substance — mucopolysaccharide — which glues the presynaptic terminal to the postsynaptic region.

The synaptic endings of axons make contact with other cells. The motor nerves that run to the major muscles may receive thousands of synaptic contacts — estimates vary between 6,000 and 30,000 — and these are distributed over the cell body and the dendrites. The motor nerves themselves end on muscle fibers in elongated structures called motor end plates. These are longer than the

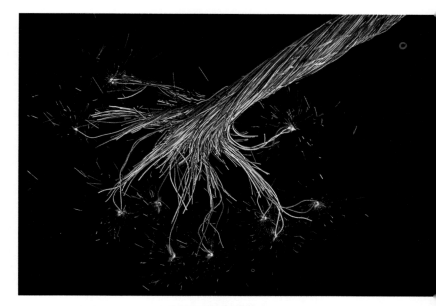

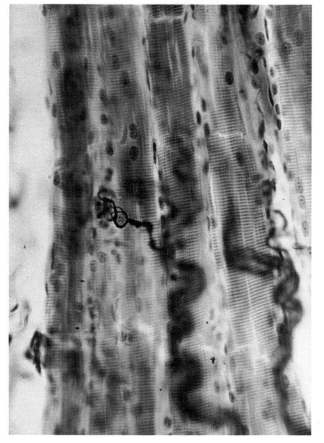

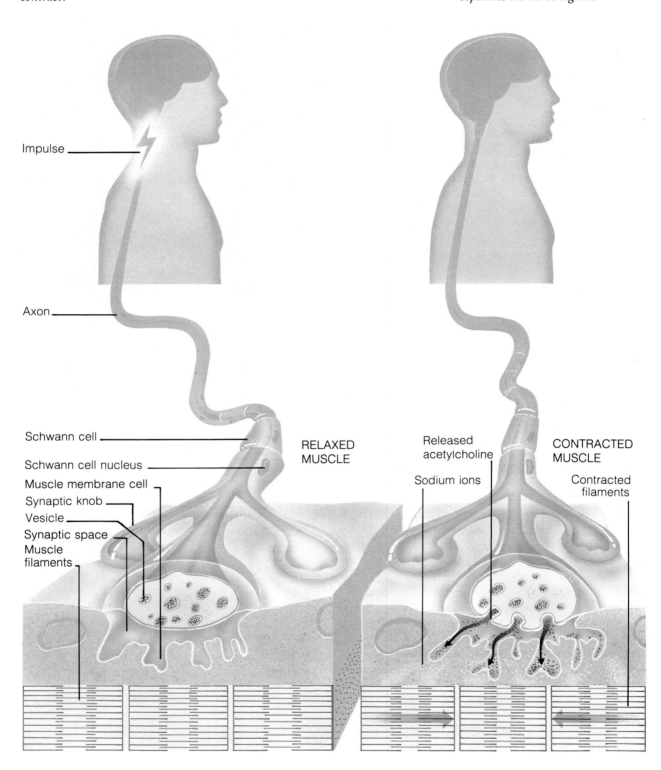

The bulges at the end of the axon of a motor nerve end on a muscle cell. An electric impulse releases acetylcholine, causing sodium to enter the muscle cell and make it contract.

In the Morse telegraph, which is conveyed in a dot-dash code, pulses of electric current are sent along a wire, just as electric impulses travel along an axon. A few milliseconds separates the nerve signals.

Impulse

Axon

Schwann cell

Schwann cell nucleus

Muscle membrane cell

Synaptic knob

Vesicle

Synaptic space

Muscle filaments

RELAXED MUSCLE

Released acetylcholine

Sodium ions

CONTRACTED MUSCLE

Contracted filaments

58

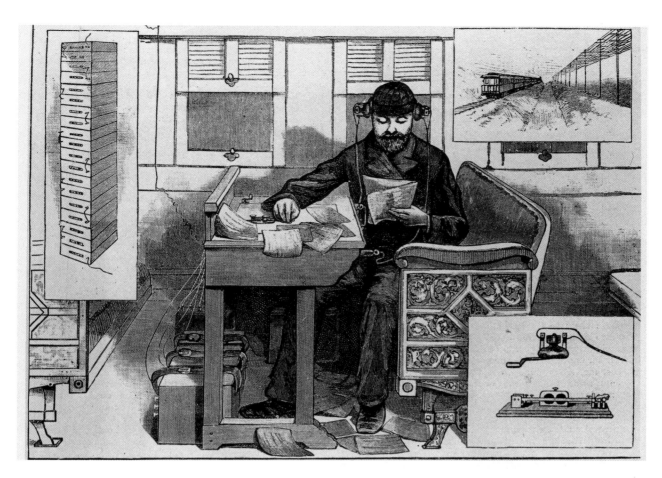

presynaptic boutons but otherwise the synaptic structure is similar. Most scientific knowledge of synaptic physiology in fact comes from studies of motor end plates.

Synaptic Transmission

When an action potential arises at a presynaptic terminal there is a delay of around one-half of a millisecond before a similar action potential is initiated in the next nerve cell or muscle. This delay is due to the nerve transmitter chemical's having to jump across the synaptic gap. In the 1920s the German-born American physiologist Otto Loewi showed that the vagus nerve to the heart releases a chemical which affects the rate of heartbeat. He called the chemical *Vagusstoff* (''vagus material'') and the biologist Henry Dale in England soon showed that it was acetylcholine, which Dale had earlier extracted from poisonous mushrooms. For their discoveries, Loewi and Dale shared the 1936 Nobel Prize in Medicine and Physiology.

In the 1930s it was supposed that acetylcholine was involved in the synapses between nerves, but it could not be detected. It then was found that the enzymes in synapses, called cholinesterases, break down the acetylcholine before it leaves the synapse. When these were inactivated, for example by the drug eserine, acetylcholine could readily be detected.

The amount of nerve transmitter released at a synapse was found to be related to the frequency of nerve impulses arriving at the presynaptic terminal. By applying minute amounts of acetylcholine to various regions of muscle fibers, Bernhard Katz and his researchers working at the University of London showed that only the synaptic region underwent depolarization. Meanwhile it was also found that impulses arriving at the presynaptic terminal caused a depolarization of the muscle membrane again in the region of the synapse, and that this depolarization preceded the propagation of action potentials over the muscle, which in turn led to muscle contraction. By recording electrical activity from inside and outside of the muscle it was found that depolarization was greatest near the end plate and that it decreased with distance from it. They were called end-plate potentials.

Studies also showed that during the end-plate potential the postsynaptic membrane increases in permeability to both sodium and potassium for one

A rifleman and a machine-gunner using identical bullets achieve different firing speeds with their different weapons. Equally, the speed of nerve impulses varies between myelinated and unmyelinated fibers.

A robot which can operate virtually on its own is controlled with electronic circuitry that resembles the human nervous system in functional concept. It involves electric currents —which is what nerve impulses are.

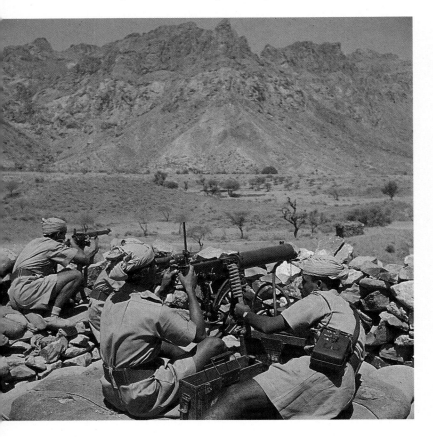

presence of vesicles in the presynaptic terminals suggests that each packet of acetylcholine corresponds to one of these vesicles, although this hypothesis is not universally accepted.

Whereas individual packets of acetylcholine apparently are released spontaneously, the arrival of an action potential at the presynaptic terminal must cause the simultaneous release of many hundreds of them. Studies using tetrodotoxin (TTX) and tetraethylammonium (TEA) to block the sodium and potassium channels respectively have shown that the release of acetylcholine depends on the movement of calcium ions into the presynaptic terminal. Calcium is at a higher concentration outside the terminal than inside, and the arrival of an impulse at the terminal appears to trigger an increase in the membrane permeability to calcium, so that this enters the terminal down its concentration gradient and somehow causes the release of transmitter. Supporting evidence has come from voltage clamp studies.

Once acetylcholine has been released from the presynaptic terminals it diffuses across the synaptic cleft to join with the receptor molecules on the postsynaptic membrane. It remains active only for one or two milliseconds before it is broken down by enzymes (acetylcholinesterases). This means that the effect of action potentials at a synapse is short-lived. The inactivated chemical is taken up by the presynaptic membrane and recycled, being re-formed into acetylcholine in the presynaptic knobs.

Postsynaptic Effects

So far only a single effect of a neurotransmitter has been considered. This is a positive or excitatory effect, that of depolarizing the postsynaptic membrane and causing excitation of the subsequent nerve cell. But synapses can also be inhibitory. Then the transmitter causes an increase in the polarization of the subsynaptic membrane, which consequently becomes more difficult to depolarize and may decrease the rate of impulse production if the cell is already active. The excitatory or inhibitory effects of a synapse depend on the transmitter and on the location of the synapse. Acetylcholine is excitatory at neuromuscular junctions but inhibitory in some parts of the autonomic system. Another trans-

to two milliseconds. The potential was therefore due to an influx of sodium, partly offset by an influx of potassium. Unlike nerves, however, in the postsynaptic membrane both ions appear to move through the same channels. So acetylcholine must somehow open the common channels, causing the change in potential which, as in nerves, is propagated electronically to neighboring regions of the muscle where it triggers action potentials and subsequent muscle contraction.

Transmitter Release

It seems that the subsynaptic membrane undergoes miniature depolarizations even in the absence of stimulation of the motor nerve. Such potentials have been shown to be due to the release of acetylcholine. These miniature end-plate potentials appear to result from the spontaneous release of discrete packets (or quanta) of transmitter molecules rather than from a random release. The

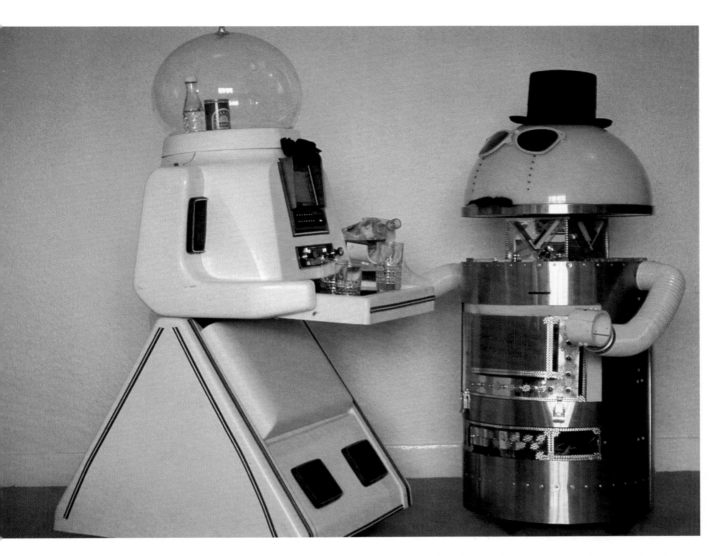

mitter, norepinephrine, can also be excitatory or inhibitory. Gamma aminobutyric acid (GABA), however, appears to be only inhibitory.

We have seen that a single nerve cell, such as a motor nerve in the ventral horn of the spinal cord, receives many hundreds of thousands of synaptic contacts; all of these may have excitatory or inhibitory effects. An impulse arriving at an excitatory synapse may depolarize the cell by only a small amount, insufficient to reach the threshold of the initial segment. But a second impulse arriving soon after the first may increase depolarization to the threshold level. The effects of the two impulses combine, a phenomenon called temporal summation. A similar effect can occur if two spatially separated synapses are excited simultaneously. The effect of either alone may be subthreshold, but together they depolarize the cell sufficiently to initiate impulse production. This is spatial summation. Of course, if the synapses have

opposite effects they may cancel out each other, or the one synapse that has the stronger effect on the cell dictates its response. Such a response, the production or suppression of impulses, therefore depends on the integration of the effects of all the active synapses. In this way, a single nerve cell can act as an integrating center for information from hundreds of thousands of other neurons and the instructions contained in that information can be regulated very precisely, in turn producing perhaps a body movement of equal precision, no more and no less what is demanded by the conscious will. Each single cell is in part responsible for the resolution of movement, or of thought, or of whatever action the neuron is contributory to.

Multiply this capacity many millions of times over for all the neurons in the central and peripheral nervous systems, and the integrating power of the nervous system clearly outweighs that of the most complex of modern computers.

Sadnefs.

Weeping.

Compafsion.

Scorn.

Horror.

Terror *or* Fright.

Anger.

Hatred *or* Jealoufy.

Defpair.

Chapter 4

Selective Systems

If the eyes are the windows of the soul, the face is the mirror of the mind, giving outward expression to inner mental states. The many different expressions the face can assume are controlled by various facial muscles, which are innervated by the cranial nerves. These nerves — the part of the peripheral nervous system that serves the head — carry commands directly from the brain. They also transmit information to it from the sense organs in the head.

The brain and the spinal cord together make up the central nervous system (CNS), although by itself the brain is the computer and control center of the body. Like a computer, the brain needs a communications network to feed information in and convey commands out, and this is the function in the body of the peripheral nervous system. Through this remarkably complex network, the brain knows much about the status of every body organ and makes constant fine adjustments to cope with a changing external and internal environment.

The peripheral nervous system transmits three main types of message, each of which can be illustrated by following through a simple, everyday act such as drinking a glass of milk. You look at the glass of milk and a sensory message travels to the brain from the eye. (Sensory messages are called afferent impulses because they carry information to the brain.) You then reach out for the glass. A motor impulse has run from your brain to the muscles in your arm and caused a voluntary movement. (Motor impulses are called efferent because they carry information away from the central nervous system.) The glass feels cold to the touch — sensory impulses again, running back to the brain from the skin, as do sensory impulses from special receptors in the joints called proprioreceptors which tell the brain exactly where your arm is. You raise the glass to your lips — you can do this even in a dark room because the proprioreceptors throughout your body tell you exactly where each part of you is in relation to another part. And as you drink the milk, many automatic responses take over — you salivate, your esophagus moves milk down to your stomach, and digestive juices. are secreted.

These last functions are in fact carried out by the automatic or autonomic nervous system, which is complex in its own right. What it does is so different from the voluntary and sensory role of the

Sensory impulses from the eyes inform the brain of the position of the glass.

Motor impulses from the brain travel to the muscles to direct the arm toward the glass.

Sensory impulses from the hand inform the brain when contact has been made with the glass.

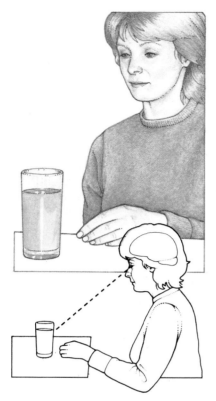

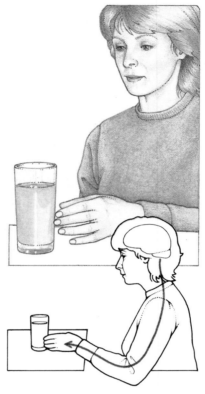

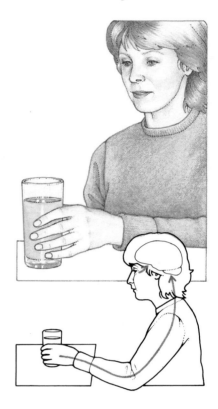

peripheral nervous system that it is considered in a separate chapter, although in reality the impulses follow the same routes. For example, if a person injures a nerve that conveys sensory messages from the hand and motor messages to it, an area becomes numb and paralyzed, but the person may also lose the ability to sweat in that area — sweating is an autonomic response.

Of the neural messages within our control, many of those that are termed "voluntary" never reach conscious awareness. And even when the body is resting or asleep afferent and efferent impulses run back and forth through the nerve fibers maintaining vital activities. You do not have to remember to breathe, even though you can pant at will or hold your breath. The skin is unable to withstand pressure for more than a couple of hours, but it is not necessary to wake up throughout the night to shift position. Receptors in the skin send messages to the muscles and you turn gently in your sleep to relieve the pressure. A person who is too weak to do this through old age or paralysis must, of course, be turned by another. But in a normal, healthy person the peripheral nervous system hums with life even though this mass of information does not

have to intrude continually on the person's conscious awareness.

An Emergency Backup System

Not every action carried out by the peripheral nervous system is under the direct control of the brain. Limited "decisions" are made by the spinal cord itself when a speedy reaction is paramount to a person's safety. Such an action takes place via a "reflex arc" which comes into play if, for example, you touch a very hot surface. Sensory messages shoot up the afferent fibers to tell the brain that pain is being felt, but at the same time the reflex arc is set off. The messages leap across special cells within the spinal cord itself and send urgent motor impulses straight back down the limb, making it withdraw swiftly from the danger. The reflex moves the hand microseconds before a voluntary message from the brain arrives via the normal routes, and these microseconds lessen the extent of damage. A split second before you are aware of pain, your arm has jerked itself out of trouble.

Spinal reflexes can be tested by a physician using a slightly different and more simple reflex, namely the stretch reflex. Inside the muscles of the body are

Motor impulses from the brain stimulate the hand to grip the glass and the arm to raise it.

Sensory impulses from the arm and eyes inform the brain of the arm's exact position as the glass is raised.

Sensory impulses from the lips inform the brain when the glass has made contact with the mouth.

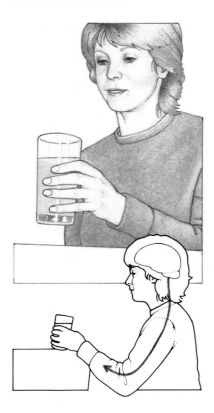
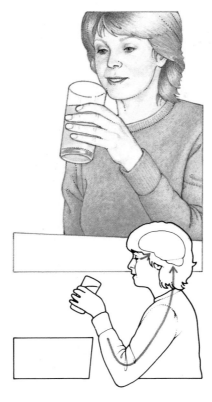
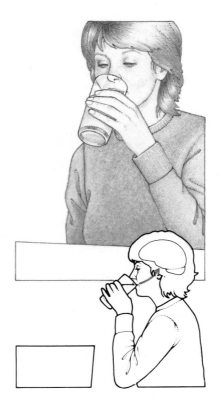

receptor cells known as muscle spindles. If the fibers in the muscle are stretched — for example, when the physician taps the tendon below the kneecap — an impulse shoots up the sensory fibers to the spinal cord, leaps across to the motor fibers and makes the muscle suddenly contract. The leg gives an involuntary jerk or kick.

All muscles in the body respond in this way when stretched, and the system safeguards them from rupture. Only certain muscle tendons are easily accessible for the physician to test, however, and the ones that might commonly be used include the ankle jerk, the triceps and biceps jerk in the arm, and the supinator reflex in the forearm. Testing these reflexes gives useful information about the condition of the spinal nerves and spinal cord.

The stretch reflex is the simplest of all spinal reflexes because the impulse passes directly from the sensory to the motor nerve. All other spinal reflexes use a kind of "stepping stone" to make the change. Anatomically, these stepping stones take the form of interneurons. Some interneurons act to cancel out other muscle contractions so that, for instance, when the quadraceps muscle at the front of the thigh needs to contract, the hamstring muscle in the back of the thigh relaxes.

The brain is not a completely innocent bystander during these processes. It influences spinal reflexes by calming them down and modifying them. Without this control from the brain the reflex becomes exaggerated and muscle tone, another function of an intact reflex system, is increased. This is tragically illustrated in the condition known as spastic palsy or paralysis in which disease or trauma affects the spinal cord and voluntary messages from the brain cannot reach the spinal nerves below the injury. The reflex arc is still intact, but the reflexes are much brisker. The person's limbs adopt a characteristic position — the arm bends at the elbow, the wrist bends, dropping the hand forwards — because the muscles that flex the limbs are stronger than the extensors.

If, however, the injury occurs on the spinal nerve itself, paralysis still affects the muscles and sensation is lost, but the muscles lose their tone and the limbs become floppy, or flaccid. There is no reflex in the muscle tendons. The dire consequences of the nervous system's operating without any inhibition are demonstrated by the

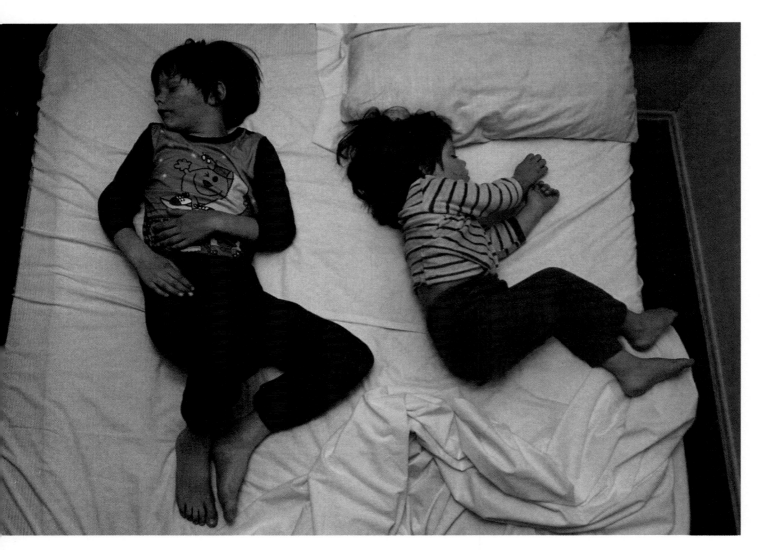

effects on the body of strychnine, a poison extracted from the seed of an East Indian shrub. It makes the victim more susceptible to stimulation, increases the reaction in the spinal motor nerves, and removes all inhibition from the spinal motor pathways so that even the slightest stimulation causes violent convulsive movements of the body. Although chemically different from strychnine, the tetanus toxin nevertheless seems to act on the body in the same way.

The Cranial Nerves

Like a map of the tributaries of a mighty river, the tiny nerve fibers from the edge of the peripheral nervous system join and interconnect until they form larger nerves which in turn connect with the spinal cord and brain.

In the human body there are 12 pairs of cranial nerves joining up with the brain, and 31 pairs of spinal nerves connecting with the spinal cord. The cranial nerves supply ordinary muscle function and sensations to the head and neck, and the spinal nerves do the same for the rest of the body. But whereas the spinal nerves carry both motor and sensory messages, the cranial nerves carry one or the other almost exclusively. The major role of the cranial nerves is to transmit messages to and from the special sense organs of sight, hearing, balance, taste and smell. Other cranial nerves form part of the autonomic nervous system and send messages that may affect organs as far distant as the small bowel and colon.

All cranial nerves pass into the skull through small holes in the bone, and it is here that they are particularly vulnerable to injury. Because of the nature of the nerves and the areas they supply, an injury to the head may produce unexpected after effects. For example, a person may lose the sense of smell following a head injury even though the nose was not damaged at all. This condition occurs

Even during sleep the nervous system does not shut down. Impulses run through the nerves to vital organs, such as the heart and lungs, and also to muscles so that the body can shift position.

Reflex arcs enable an almost immediate reaction in certain situations—for example, when touching a hot object such as the roast chestnut that the boy finds too hot to handle.

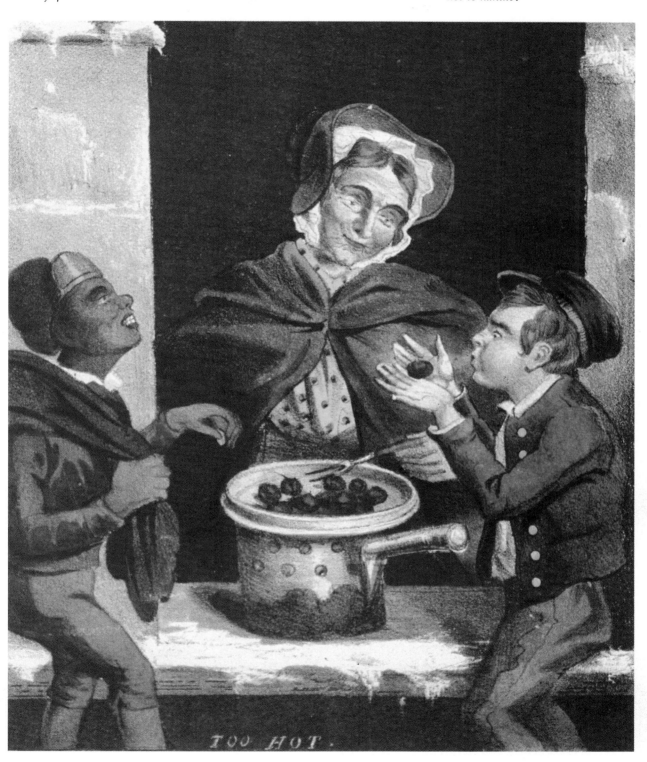

TOO HOT.

because the olfactory nerves responsible for the most primitive special sense, that of smell, have been damaged, usually permanently.

The optic nerves, which take messages from the eyes to the brain, can also produce bewildering visual defects if damaged by trauma or disease. It is only through detailed understanding of the complicated anatomy of the visual system that the physician can diagnose the exact location of the damage. For example, a tumor pressing on the optic nerve behind the right eye blinds the eye; if, however, it presses on the nerve on the right side after it has emerged from the junction of the two nerves (the optic chiasma), both eyes partially lose their capacity for visual perception.

The oculomotor, trochlear and abducens nerves help to move the eyeball, and the trigeminal nerves supply the face's sensation. The facial nerves connect with some of the tongue's taste glands and the muscles of facial expression. Sometimes a facial nerve suffers a temporary injury, causing muscle weakness on just one side of the face. The eye and corner of the mouth droop, the cheek is flaccid, the mouth is incontinent and the person drools. The condition is known as Bell's palsy.

The cochlear or auditory nerves convey sound impulses from the inner ear, and the vestibular portions of the auditory nerves convey the sensation of balance from the semicircular canals in the inner ear. The glossopharyngeal nerves take other taste sensations to the brain from the tongue and help to supply salivary glands through their autonomic nerves.

The vagus nerves are the longest cranial nerves of all, and their influence is felt in regions of the body as remote from the brain as the thorax and abdomen. One area they reach is the stomach, where they control the secretion of stomach acid. If the stomach is producing too much acid, which in turn is eroding the delicate wall of the duodenum and causing an ulcer, a surgeon may cut the nerve (an operation called a vagotomy), which reduces the acid flow and accordingly helps the ulcer to begin to heal.

The accessory nerves supply the two large muscles in front of and behind the neck which support the head, and the hypoglossal nerves supply the muscles of the tongue.

Pathways from the Spinal Cord

The spinal cord lies within the vertebral column, the bony tube made up of vertebrae stacked one upon the other, which surrounds and protects it. Fibrous pads (intervertebral disks) containing a semifluid jellylike substance cushioning the bones lie between the vertebrae and act as shock absorbers. They make up just less than a third of the height of the vertebral column in a young person.

The spinal nerves lead off the spinal cord in pairs, one on either side while still inside the vertebral column. Each nerve leaves the cord as two roots, one in front of the other. The one at the front is called the ventral root and transmits only motor impulses. The back one, the dorsal root, carries the impulses of sensation. The two roots join up again inside the vertebral column.

That the dorsal root carried sensation and the ventral root carried motor impulses was originally suspected as early as 1811 by a Scotsman named Sir Charles Bell. One of his assistants demonstrated Bell's experiments to a Frenchman, François Magendie, who in 1822 published his own findings — to the fury of Sir Charles, who then vociferously claimed that it was he who had been the first to make the discovery. The subsequent controversy lasted for many years, but it is now accepted that Magendie made the full discovery even though Bell's early work was its forerunner.

Before the dorsal and ventral roots are traced down inside the vertebral column to their exit hole, one more interesting difference between the two deserves to be noted. Spinal nerves consist of bunches of nerve cells, and their characteristic spaghetti-strand appearance is made up from the bunching of the axons — the long, thin parts of the cell. But nerve cells also have a nucleus. The nuclei of the nerve cells of the ventral root lie in one of the bulges, or horns, of the spinal cord itself and are called anterior horn cells. This is not the case with the dorsal root. Here the cell bodies with their nuclei gather together in a clump which sticks up above the dorsal root like a bud on the branch of a tree. This clump is the dorsal root ganglion.

Exit from the Spinal Cord

The re-fused nerve containing motor and sensory fibers winds down inside the spinal column

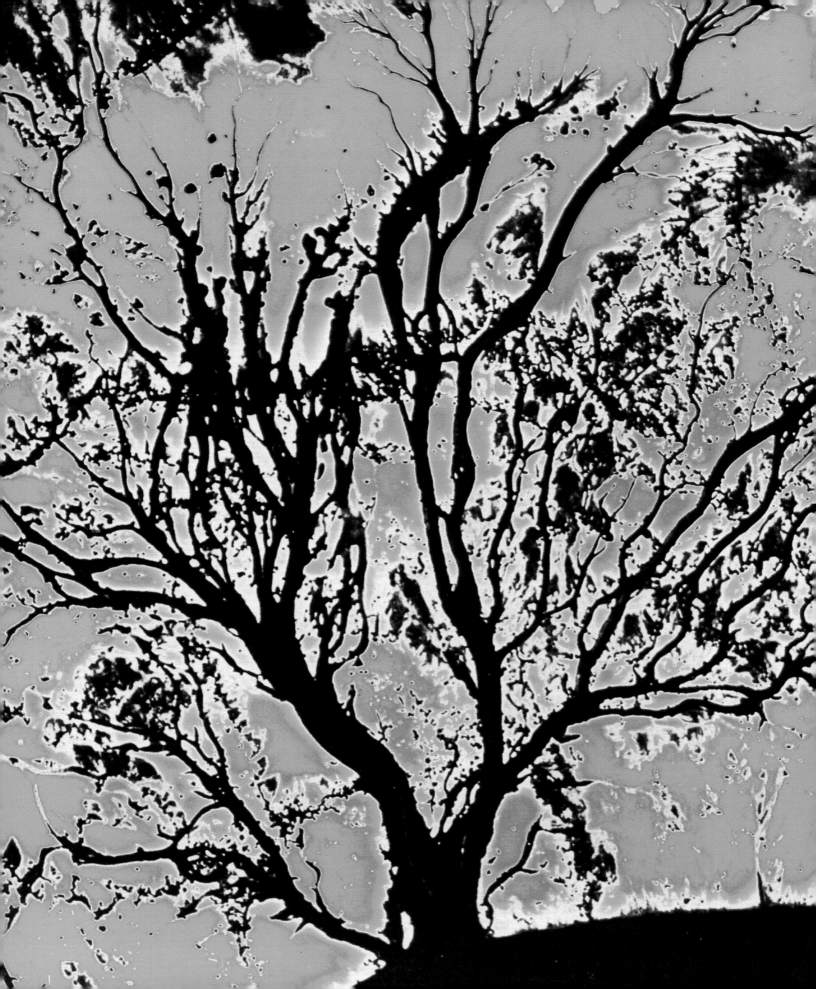

In the center of the photomicrograph below is a neuromuscular spindle (magnified about 750 times and shown in cross section), a stretch receptor found in skeletal muscles. These receptors are involved in the regulation of muscle tone and in the control of precision movements, such as the fine hand movements made by a surgeon performing a delicate operation (exploring the spinal cord in the bottom photograph).

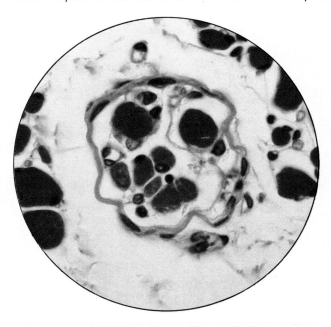

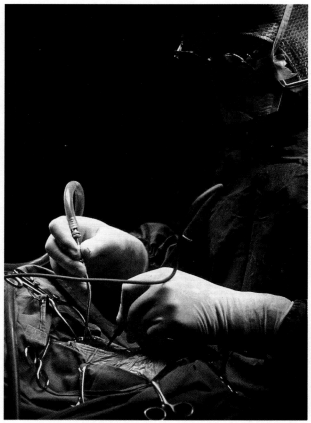

alongside the cord itself until it reaches its exit hole, or intervertebral foramen. The spinal cord is actually shorter than the spinal column; the nerves at the top come out of the spinal column almost at a right angle, but the farther down the spinal cord a nerve emerges, the longer the journey for the nerve to its exit foramen. It is as if the bony canal has outgrown the spinal cord and left the end of it behind. The spinal nerves that exit from the lumbar, sacral and coccygeal levels have to travel down the lower part of the spinal canal as a mass of nerves, and because they look like the tail of a horse they are called, in Latin, *cauda equina*.

When the nerve reaches its exit foramen it comes out from the protection of the spinal column. Here it again splits into two separate strands, but this time the function of sensory and motor impulses are equally apportioned to each strand. The smaller strand, the one at the back, is called the posterior primary branch or ramus. This carries motor and sensory impulses to the skin and muscles of the back. The front strand is larger and is called the anterior primary ramus. It has to be larger because it supplies not only the skin and muscles of the front of the body, but also most of the "plexuses," large bunches of interconnecting nerves.

The Dermatomes of the Skin

Many of the anterior primary rami run around the front of the body parallel to the ribs. Each ramus supplies the muscle and a single strip of skin called a dermatome, and many of these radiate around the body in a pattern rather like a striped body stocking, dipping down lower at the front than the back. For example, the spinal nerve from the center of the back supplies an area of skin which includes the navel. The dermatomes overlap a little, so that cutting of one spinal nerve leaves an area of skin less sensitive but not completely numb.

The stripes on the body stocking change when they reach the limbs. Instead of horizontal hoops, the pattern elongates into vertical stripes that run down the limbs. The legs, and their large muscles, need generous supplies of motor impulses, and the arms — and particularly the hand and fingers — require a nerve supply large enough to accommodate their huge sensory input and to control their delicate movements.

François Magendie and Sir Charles Bell

War of Nerves

In a period of great political upheaval and marked nationalism the Scottish physician Sir Charles Bell (1774–1842) and the French physiologist François Magendie (1783–1855) had a battle of their own.

In 1811 Bell published *Idea of a New Anatomy of the Brain* in which he outlined his theory that the anterior nerve roots of the spinal cord carry impulses to the muscles and give rise to motion while the posterior nerve roots carry impulses to the brain that are interpreted as sensation. It was hailed by his peers as a "new Magna Carta of neurology," which gives a vivid impression of the invigorating impact it had on scientific thought. When, eleven years later, Magendie provided conclusive evidence for Bell's observations, a controversy was sparked off as to whom credit for the discovery belonged which was to be resolved only in the first half of this century, with the Frenchman taking the victor's laurels.

The early careers of the two men were similar. They both rose rapidly in their chosen field of anatomy, holding a succession of prestigious posts, before deciding that physiology was where their main interest lay. They were of one mind in

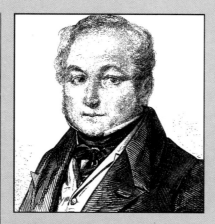

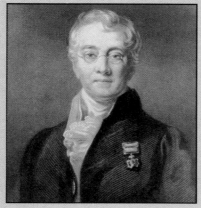

rejecting the nonempirical methodology of the day and turned instead to meticulous dissection and experimentation to unravel the intricacies of the nervous system.

Temperamentally, however, they were worlds apart. Bell was described as being "distinguished by unpretending amenity, and simplicity of manners and deportment." Magendie's

dogmatic and fiery character, on the other hand, made him numerous enemies. A close colleague was not alone in thinking that "his cult of experimentation misled the physiologist, effaced the teacher, and suppressed the doctor."

Magendie's use of vivisection—though he was not averse to experimenting on himself occasionally—added to his unsavory reputation and tended to obscure the many benefits that resulted from his work. He was instrumental in introducing morphine and strychnine into medical practice. And his research into nutrition and the stress he placed on the importance of protein came at a much needed stage in France's history, when revolution had stripped the country of its resources and caused a scarcity of food.

Meanwhile the Bell–Magendie debate raged on. But the heat generated by the supporters of each protagonist created a climate conducive to further research and Magendie's enormously talented pupil, Claude Bernard, contributed much that has led to our present knowledge of physiology—so that somehow out of chaos and dissension came order and understanding.

71

The sensory and motor requirements of the thorax and abdomen are satisfied by a pair of thoracic spinal nerves for each dermatome. But this is not enough for the limbs, where instead spinal nerves join up into networks of fibers before branching off down the limbs; these networks are called the plexuses.

There are three major plexuses — cervical, brachial and lumbosacral — made up from the front spinal nerves (anterior primary rami). The branches at the back, the posterior primary rami, are not involved at all.

Nerve Supplies to the Arms

The cervical plexus, which lies in the neck, collects and integrates two spinal nerves, then sends out re-sorted fibers to the skin of the head and neck. One important nerve that emerges from the cervical plexus is the phrenic nerve, which travels down to the diaphragm and is the main nerve used for breathing. In the days before antibiotics, when tuberculosis was a common and much feared disease, the lung could be rested by paralyzing one side of the diaphragm. This was effected by crushing the phrenic nerve during a relatively simple operation in the neck.

The brachial plexus lies at the root of the neck behind the clavicle and is made up of three or four cervical spinal nerves. The plexus crosses and intermingles the nerves before sending them down the arm intimately wrapped around the main blood vessels. Because the nerves of the arm are located in a virtually identical position in all persons, an injury to a particular nerve always produces the same signs. For example, dislocation of the shoulder can damage the axillary nerve and produce an area of numbness over the shoulder, whereas a fracture of the humerus in the upper arm can damage the radial nerve (which is wrapped around this bone) causing weakness of wrist extension, or "wrist drop." The large median nerve has much to do with the movement and feeling in the fingers and hand, and in order to reach these areas it passes through a tight canal — a carpal tunnel — in the wrist. If the nerve gets trapped in it the fingers tingle and the thumb weakens, a condition known as carpal tunnel syndrome.

Another common injury to a nerve of the peripheral nervous system is one of which many people have experience. The ulnar nerve gives sensory impulses over the little finger and part of the third finger. It lies on the bone just below the skin on the inner side of the elbow, and when the "funny bone" is knocked it is the ulnar nerve that causes tingling and pain, not the bone at all.

Nerve Supplies to the Legs

The lumbosacral plexus gathers in eight spinal nerves before sending out a mass of nerves down the legs. Many join up to form the largest single nerve in the body, the sciatic nerve, which is about the thickness of an adult's little finger.

The huge sciatic nerve snakes its way down through the buttock, delivering some of its motor and sensory impulses to the hamstring muscle at the back of the leg. Then it divides and thins out to supply the calf and foot. Although it seems to be protected by a mass of muscle, the sciatic nerve can be damaged in the buttock itself by a badly placed injection into the muscles. The pain felt when this nerve is injured is called sciatica, and is typically caused by pressure on a nerve as it leaves the spinal column. The pressure may be caused by a protrusion of an intervertebral disk, a condition familiarly known as a "slipped disk."

The Tracts of the Spinal Cord

A spinal nerve transmits both sensory and motor messages for a particular part of the body, as we have seen, so at any one time it may have passing through it temperature sensations and light touch sensations as well as messages to the muscles from the brain giving voluntary commands for movement. This mixture of information is transmitted along the same route. However, once the nerve feeds the messages into the spinal cord itself, they are sorted, separated and then streamed into groups of nerve fibers called tracts. For example, one tract carries sensations of pain and temperature, another carries those of light touch or tells the brain exactly where each limb is in relation to the rest of the body. Yet another carries voluntary movement messages down from the brain. This principle is the fundamental difference between the peripheral nervous system and the central nervous system. In the peripheral system all the messages

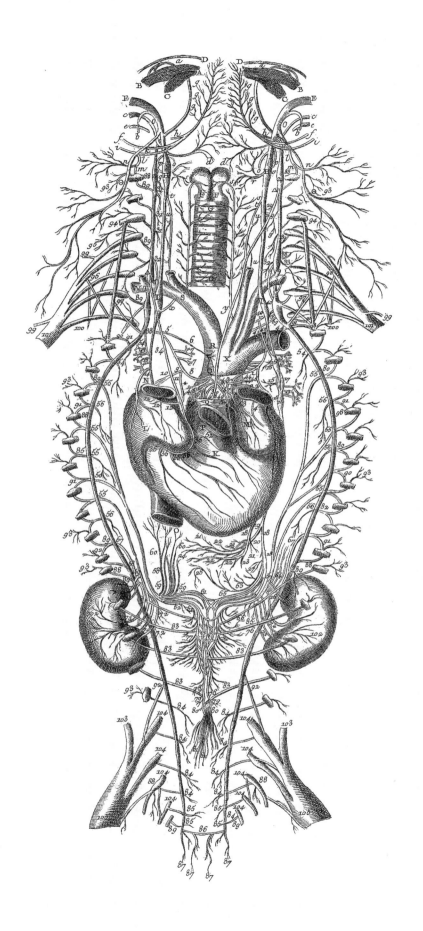

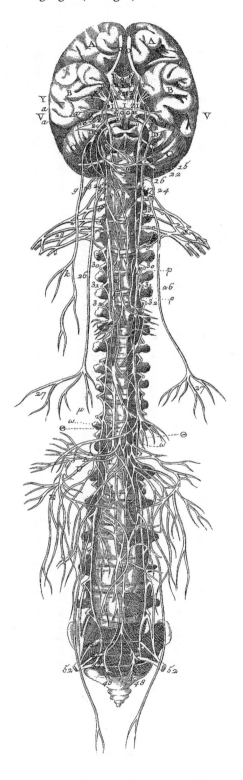

By making meticulous dissections, eighteenth-century anatomists gradually unraveled the structure of the nervous system. Today electron microscopes reveal the finest detail of ganglia (far right).

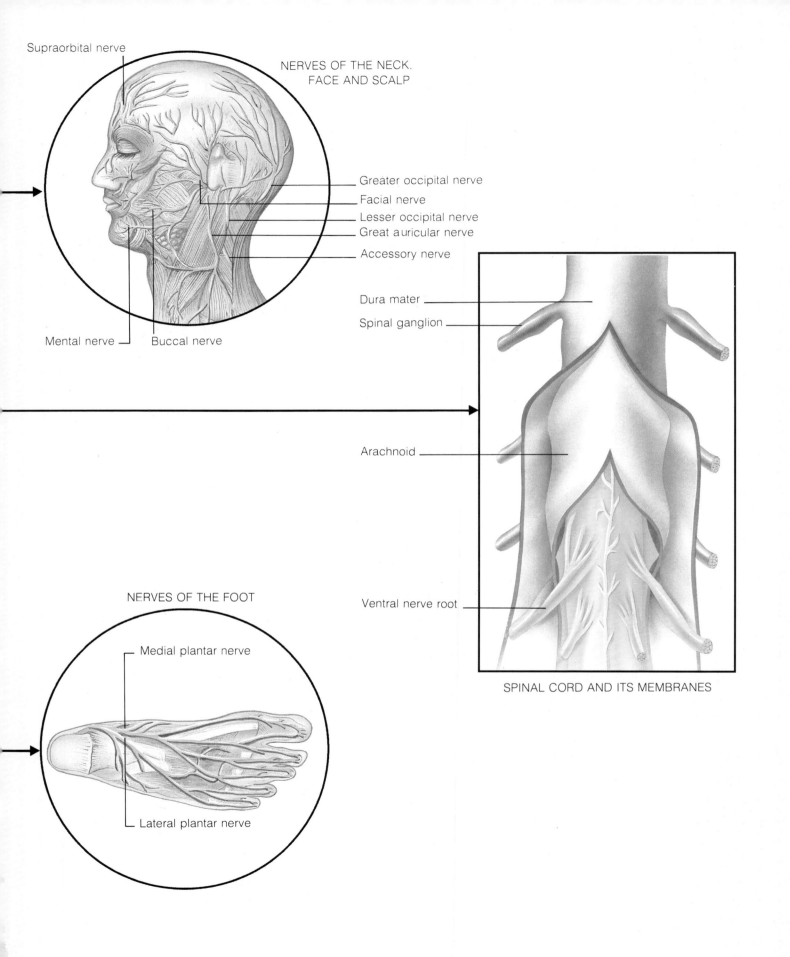

Supraorbital nerve

NERVES OF THE NECK,
FACE AND SCALP

Greater occipital nerve
Facial nerve
Lesser occipital nerve
Great auricular nerve
Accessory nerve

Mental nerve — Buccal nerve

Dura mater
Spinal ganglion

Arachnoid

Ventral nerve root

NERVES OF THE FOOT

Medial plantar nerve

Lateral plantar nerve

SPINAL CORD AND ITS MEMBRANES

The nervous system forms an intricate mesh that runs throughout the body, linking not only the major organs but also individual sensory receptors (such as touch receptors in the skin) into a complex information gathering, processing and transmitting network. Highly sophisticated and fast-acting, the nervous system enables us to respond almost instantaneously to external or internal stimuli.

The nervous system has two main parts: the central nervous system (which consists of the brain and spinal cord), and the peripheral nervous system (which is comprised of all the other nerves, including the autonomic ones). This illustration shows the anatomical relationship between the central nervous system and the main peripheral nerves (excluding those of the autonomic nervous system).

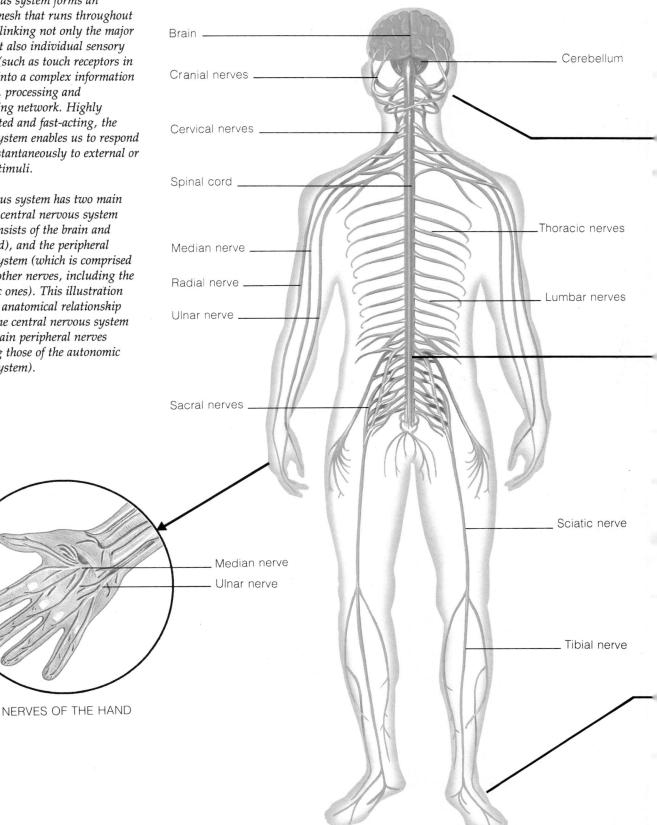

Brain

Cranial nerves

Cervical nerves

Spinal cord

Median nerve

Radial nerve

Ulnar nerve

Sacral nerves

Cerebellum

Thoracic nerves

Lumbar nerves

Sciatic nerve

Tibial nerve

Median nerve

Ulnar nerve

NERVES OF THE HAND

PERIPHERAL SYSTEM

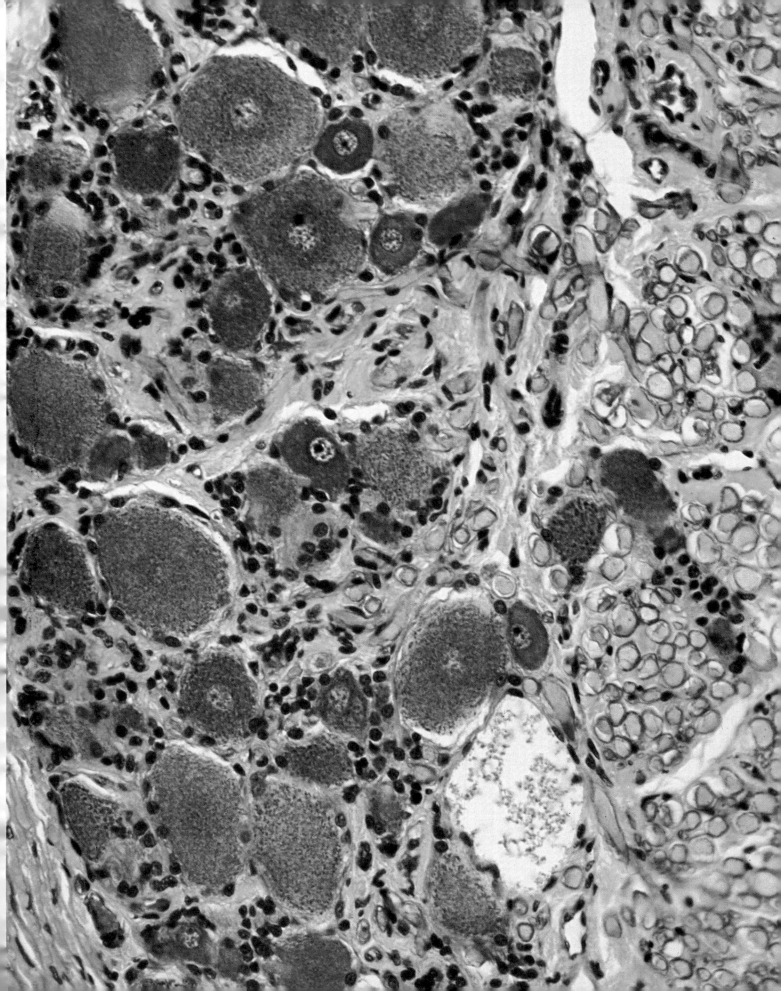

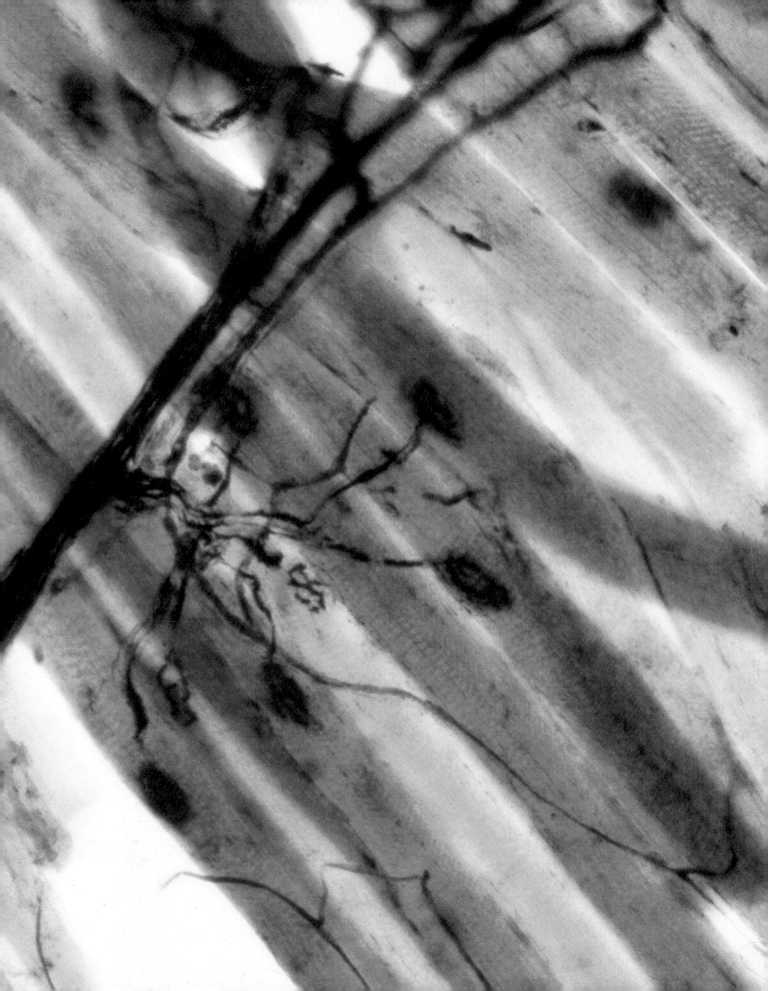

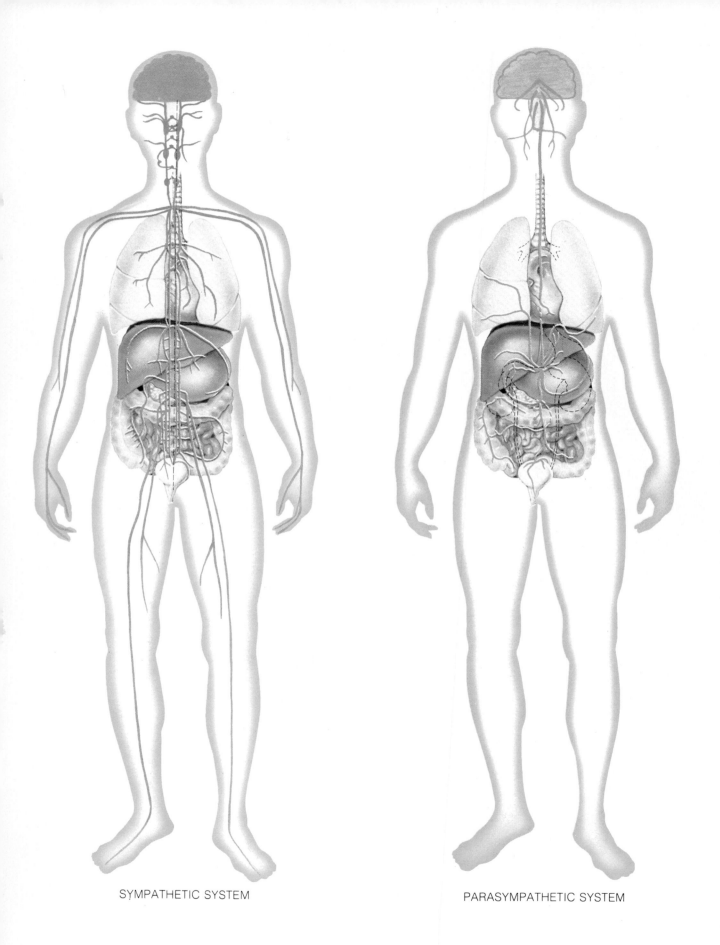

SYMPATHETIC SYSTEM

PARASYMPATHETIC SYSTEM

The parasympathetic system is one of the two divisions of the autonomic nervous system. It consists of long preganglionic fibers in the facial, glossopharyngeal, oculomotor and vagus cranial nerves (arising from the base of the brain and the brainstem), and in nerves from the second, third and fourth sacral segments of the lower spinal cord; it also includes numerous outlying ganglia (mostly situated near or within the end organs), and short postganglionic fibers. The facial nerve supplies the salivary and tear glands; the glossopharyngeal, the mouth; the oculomotor, the eye; and the vagus, most of the visceral organs. The sacral parasympathetics innervate the bladder, sex organs and part of the intestines.

The sympathetic system is the other of the two divisions of the autonomic nervous system. It consists of short preganglionic fibers arising from the twelve thoracic (chest) and first three lumbar (lower back) segments of the spinal cord; a paired chain of ganglia running alongside the spinal cord; several outlying ganglia; and long postganglionic fibers from the ganglia to end organs. Generally, the sympathetic system innervates the same organs as does the parasympathetic system (the adrenal glands are the principal exception, being supplied only by sympathetic nerves). But the two systems have opposite effects; for example, sympathetic stimulation increases the heartrate whereas parasympathetic stimulation decreases it.

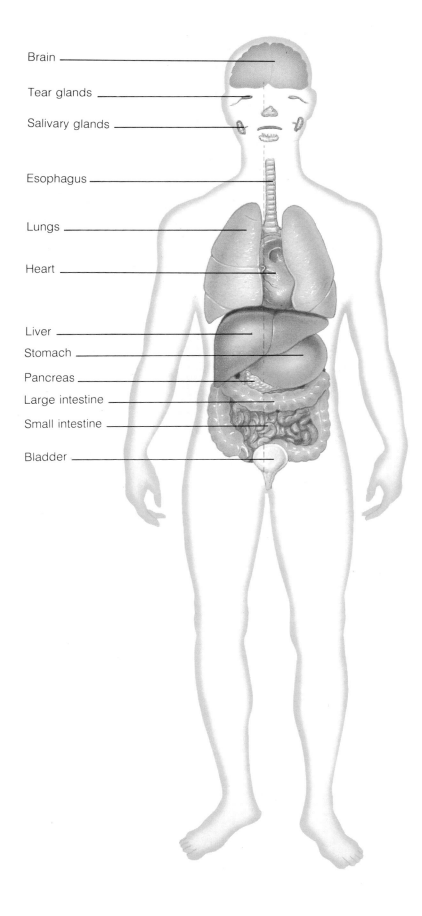

Brain

Tear glands

Salivary glands

Esophagus

Lungs

Heart

Liver

Stomach

Pancreas

Large intestine

Small intestine

Bladder

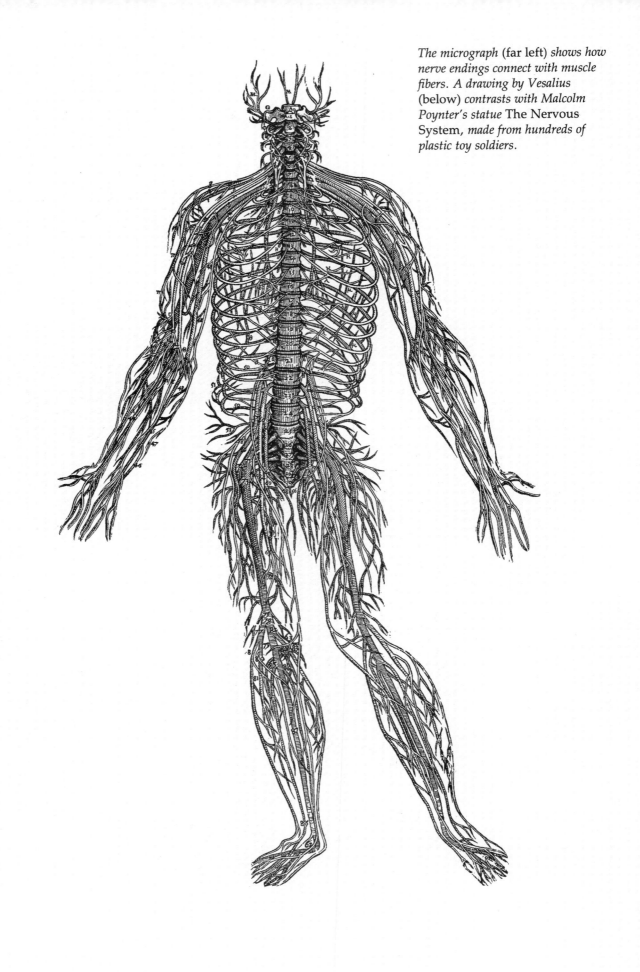

The micrograph (far left) shows how nerve endings connect with muscle fibers. A drawing by Vesalius (below) contrasts with Malcolm Poynter's statue The Nervous System, *made from hundreds of plastic toy soldiers.*

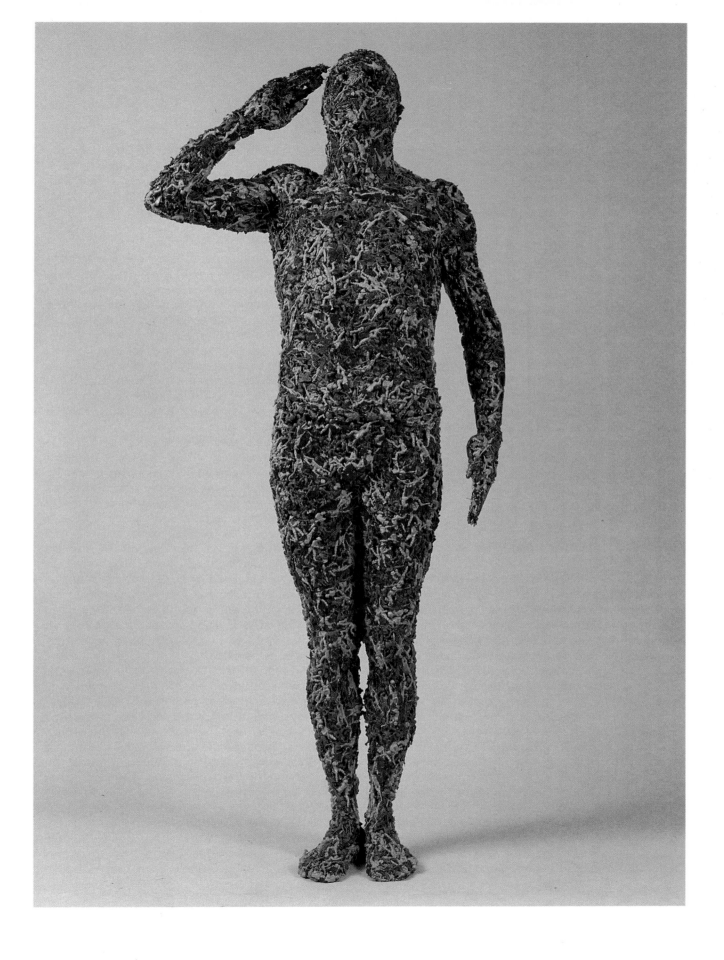

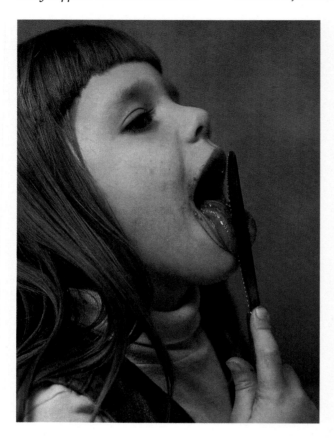

there is some banding. Fibers destined for the cervical spinal nerves lie in the band next to those destined for the thoracic spinal nerves, and they peel off as they leave the cord like individual airplanes from a formation.

Receptors in the Skin

The brain depends upon a battery of receptors to keep it in constant touch with all aspects of the body and the environment. Energy sources that stimulate receptors vary tremendously — sound waves for hearing, light energy for sight, and heat energy for temperature reception, for instance. Receptors, in their turn, are just as varied. However, there is only one way in which all this information can be relayed to the brain, and that is by way of an electrical impulse fed into the peripheral nervous system and transmitted to the central nervous system.

To study the system in action, it is pertinent to consider one single impulse which has started in a receptor in the skin, and follow its journey from the peripheral nervous system to the central nervous system. The whole is like a relay race involving several different runners.

A sensation of temperature is picked up by a receptor in the skin and this sets off the impulse which begins to travel up the axon of the nerve cell. This nerve cell is called the first order neuron. The impulse rushes along like a relay runner past the cell's body in the dorsal root ganglion, then on to the spinal cord itself. The runner must now pass on the nerve impulse to the second order neuron which lies in the "wing tip" of the butterfly-sectioned spinal cord. This area of the cord is the substantia gelatinosa, and here the impulse is handed on for the second leg of the race.

The long arm (axon) of the nerve cell crosses the "running track" of the spinal cord and the runner gets into a "lane" on the opposite side, a bundle of nerves called the lateral spinothalamic tract in the white matter of the spinal cord. The impulse is rushed up this tract until it reaches the thalamus (the main sensory relay nucleus of the brain), where it is handed over for the last time.

The distance each runner covers changes according to which impulse is being carried. Temperature, pain, and fine touch sensations from the skin give

are jumbled, whereas in the central system they are sorted and streamed.

The spinal cord, like the brain, is made up of two main types of tissue, gray matter and white matter. Imagine that the spinal cord has been cut across horizontally and that you are looking down on the cut. The gray matter looks like the wings of a butterfly surrounded by white matter. The white matter consists of nerve fibers in their tracts, covered in fatty myelin. The gray matter is made up of the cell bodies of the nerve cells.

The proportion of gray matter to white matter in the spinal cord changes, depending on the distance from the brain. Think of a railway network. The nearer you are to a main station the more railway lines there are — the same applies to the mass of tracts squeezing together as they near the brain. At the other end of the spinal cord a similar horizontal cut would reveal a large area of gray matter framed by a thin coat of white matter. Within these tracts

A detail from the Flemish artist Jan Brueghel's **The Distinguished Visitor** *shows, among the profusion of activities in this scene of peasant life, a child and a mother and her baby warming themselves by the fire.*

Heat from any source is dectected by temperature-sensitive nerve endings (thermoreceptors) in the skin. These send ''heat'' impulses to the spinal cord, which conducts the impulses to the brain.

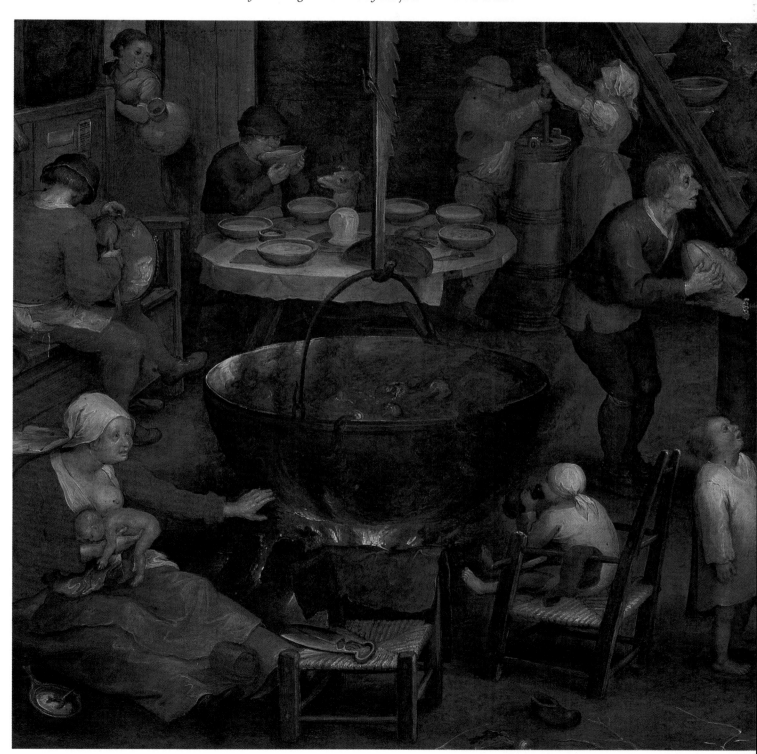

the first and second runner a long race, but the third runner has an easy, short sprint. Often, however, it is the first runner that has to do the marathon run, and the second and third runners who have the short sprint.

Once the impulse has been handed over for the last time (to an appropriate area of the sensory cortex), that part of the brain must translate the message, package a command up in another impulse, and send it from the motor cortex to the motor nerves of the spinal cord, and finally back to the muscles. The nerve cells used to take the message back down the spinal cord may be up to a yard long, so only two runners are needed to relay it. The first runner changes lanes and rushes down the opposite corticospinal tract where it passes the impulse across to the spinal nerve for the last stage of the journey.

The lane-changing of the impulses occurs at different levels in the central nervous system, but no matter where the change happens, all impulses from the left side of the body cross over at some stage to reach the opposite side of the brain. Thus the right side of the brain is responsible for the sensory and motor functions of the left side of the body, and if a person is right-handed, the left side of the brain is the dominant one. This explains why a stroke in the right side of the brain causes left-sided paralysis.

The spinal tracts have been studied extensively and detailed knowledge of their pathways now exists. A great deal of the pioneering work in this field was carried out during the early nineteenth century by a Frenchman named Charles Brown-Séquard. He discovered that if the spinal cord was cut partly through, a consistent pattern of abnormalities resulted. On the side of the damage the muscles went into a spastic paralysis and the senses of light touch and joint position were lost, but on the opposite side of the body the ability to feel pain or temperature changes was lost. This pattern of sensory abnormalities following hemisection of the spinal cord is still referred to as the Brown-Séquard syndrome.

Tertiary syphilis is now a rare condition because the disease can be cured in its early stages. A formerly bewildering symptom of the disease, however, was the fact that the sufferer was unable to judge when the foot was about to touch the ground, and so walked with a strange, plonking step. The skin was numb to a light touch, but felt pain and temperature as accurately as would a healthy person's. This effect is now understood: the dorsal tracts which transmit touch and position sense were affected by the disease; other tracts were not involved.

Some receptors, such as those in the nose, stop giving impulses if the stimulation from outside is constant; after a while the sensation disappears altogether. For example, a shirt made of rough material is at first intolerably itchy against the skin. After about half an hour or so the feeling fades until the shirt is comfortable. The phenomenon is called adaptation. Another example is a ticking clock which at first is insistently loud but after a time becomes quite inaudible.

Electrical impulses generated by receptors travel along nerves which vary in diameter, length and the thickness of the myelin insulation. Large, well-myelinated fibers conduct impulses faster than small, unmyelinated fibers. The fastest conducting fibers are Alpha types which transmit impulses that come from receptors in the joints. These receptors tell the brain where the limbs are in relation to the body and are called proprioreceptors. Impulses transmitted more slowly include touch and pressure, pain and temperature. Some painful sensations are sent up to the brain by way of very fine nerve fibers, thus the impulse moves comparatively slowly. If you jump off a wall and land heavily on your feet, you feel the pain about a second after your feet hit the ground.

Messages to the Muscles

All the motor impulses coming from the brain and relayed by spinal motor neurons are destined for the muscles. Each spinal motor nerve ends in a group of muscle fibers, and the nerve cell along with its bundles of muscle fibers is called a motor unit. The number of muscle fibers in a motor unit varies considerably depending on the part of the body it moves. The eyeball muscles have a nerve cell to supply every five or six muscle fibers, whereas the large power muscles in the thigh may demand that a single nerve cell supply as many as 150 muscle fibers.

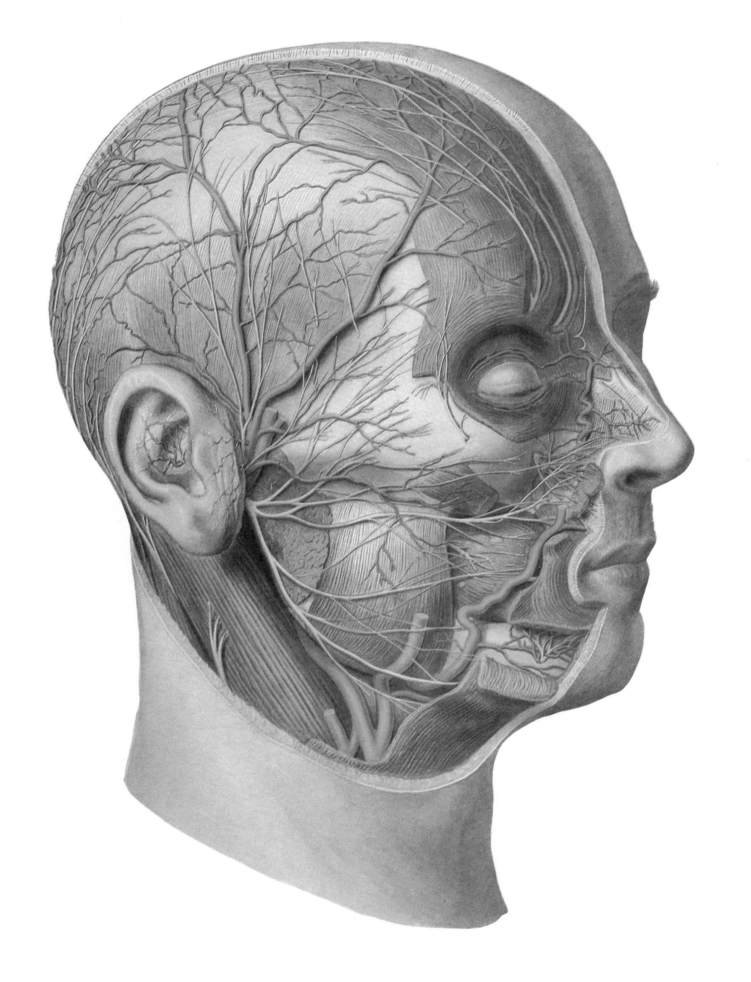

At the end of each motor nerve is a special structure called an end plate. When the nerve impulse from the central nervous system arrives at the end plate, the muscle contracts although there is no direct electrical contact between the nerve and the muscle. The impulse is passed to the muscle in small vesicles (packets of chemicals) and it is these that make the muscle contract. The process can actually be timed — it takes about one thousandth of a second.

It is this process which comes under attack when certain chemicals enter the bloodstream. Neuroblockers such as curare stop the vesicles from arriving at their receptors. The toxin released by the botulism germ in a form of food poisoning is also a neuroblocker, but in this case the chemical in the vesicles is not released.

Chemical transmission does not happen only at the motor end plate, it occurs at other junctions or synapses too. But just as these chemical means are used by neurons to pass on a nerve impulse, there are neurons in the system which use the same chemical method to restrict or halt the impulse's passage. In fact, connected with the axons of many other cells, both facilitating and inhibitory neurons may act on a single nerve cell at the same time and thus regulate its activity to a remarkable degree of precision. It is this careful balancing that decides whether or how an impulse is transmitted.

Balance is the key to the successful working of the peripheral nervous system. Everything is finely tuned, from the tone in the muscles right down to the miniature chemical transmissions playing one against the other to produce the exactly appropriate impulse. This balancing and juggling of impulses, of senses and commands, continues without our ever stopping to think, when we reach for that glass of milk, how many intricate and complicated processes are acting together to perform one simple act. Conversely, it is sometimes with concentration and willpower that we try to be precise in our actions, and again it is thanks to the peripheral nervous system that we may, perhaps to some extent, succeed. Precision of movement, or of thought — in concert pianists or brain surgeons, for example — may be extreme. Yet the capacity for it is in all of us.

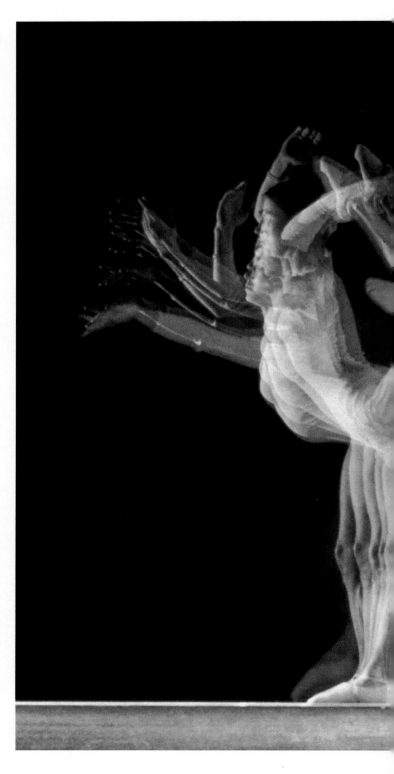

Performing acrobatics on a narrow beam needs superb balance and coordination. Such a feat requires a continual flow of sensory information to the brain from the ears (which contain the organs of balance) and proprioceptors (which inform the brain of the exact position of the limbs) in the joints. The peripheral motor nerves are also essential to transmit "movement" commands from brain to muscles.

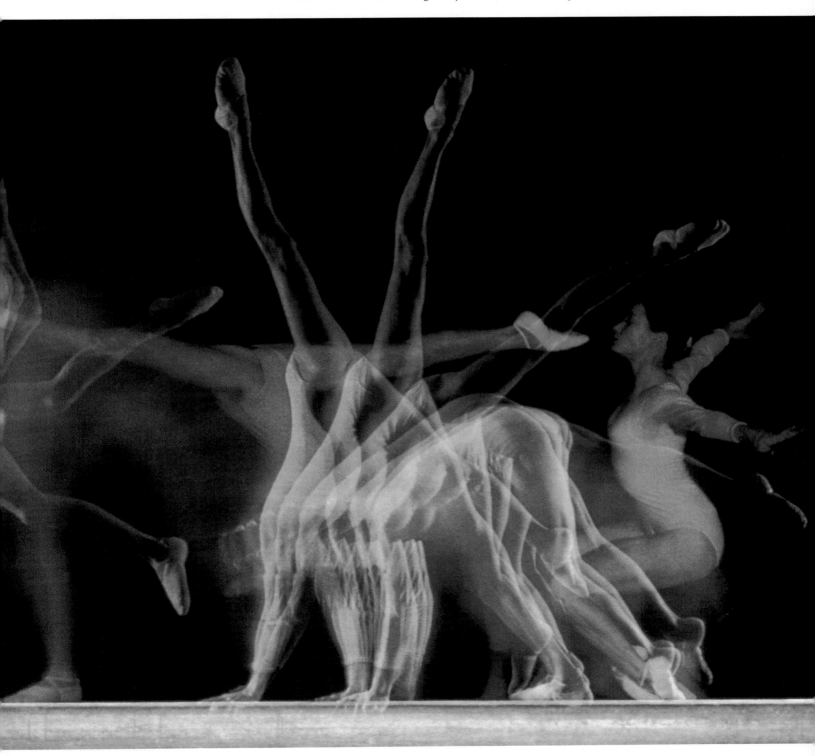

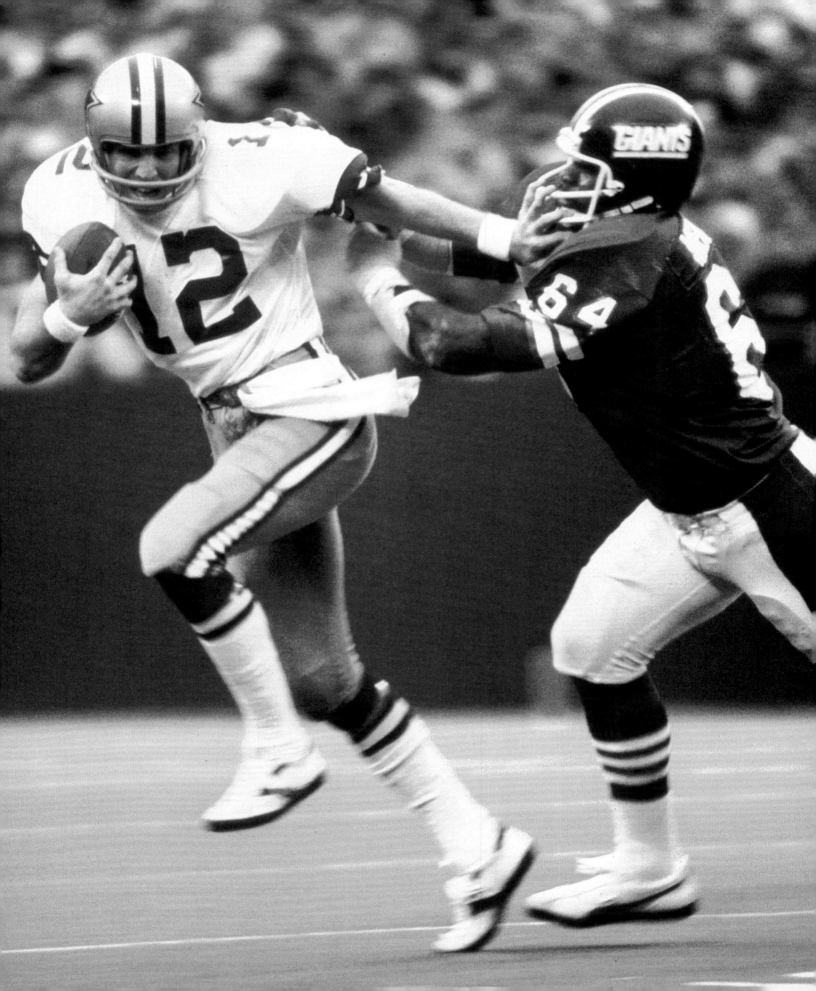

Chapter 5

Automatic Actions

When the body needs more oxygen, breathing becomes faster. When more blood needs to be pumped around the body, the heart beats faster. After a meal is eaten, the food is digested. All these things occur automatically and although you may sometimes be aware that they are happening, they are not in the control of the conscious will. They are involuntary responses designed to maintain an internal stability and to allow the body to meet the demands of its interactions with the external environment.

Consider strenuous exercise, for example. The brain tells the skeletal muscles to work, but the muscles are not able to sustain the exercise unless provided with the extra fuel and oxygen required. Respiration speeds up, the heart rate increases, vessels delivering blood to the muscles dilate, and stored glucose is released. The end result is that more oxygenated blood flows to the working muscles so that the fuel can be "burned" to provide energy for muscle contraction. Of course, efficiency is not 100 per cent (about 25 per cent for muscles), so a lot of energy is wasted and released as heat. This raises the temperature of the body and more involuntary responses have to be made to reduce body heat: sweating begins and blood is shunted via the skin so that heat can be lost from the body surface.

A similar situation exists when the body is under threat. Everyone has experienced a degree of fright or threat which has made the heart pound, the mouth dry, the hairs prickle at the back of the neck, and the eyes seemingly pop out of their sockets. This is all part of the fight-or-flight response by which the body prepares itself for a defense reaction.

These examples really are only the tip of a very complex iceberg. All the body's internal functions — from mucus secretion in the nose and the level of calcium in blood and bone, to the caliber of blood vessels in the big toe — are regulated and

Many bodily functions are controlled automatically by the autonomic nervous system so that the body can adapt to changing conditions without the need for conscious decisions. For example, during exercise — such as playing football or any other strenuous sport — the body requires more energy, so the autonomic nervous system responds automatically to modify the body's metabolism to meet this need.

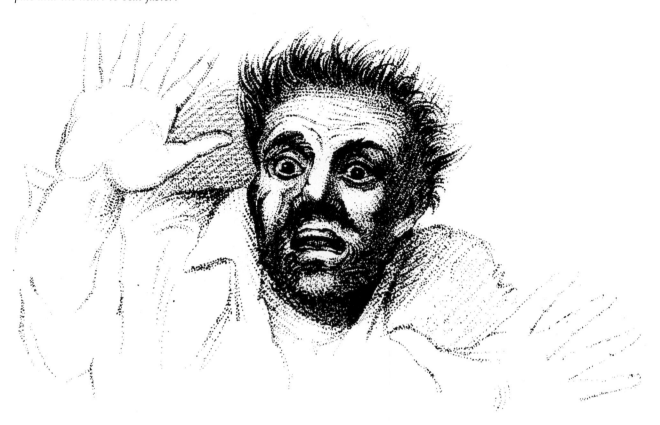

coordinated by two systems: the chemical messages (or hormones) of the endocrine system and the electrical messages of the autonomic nervous system. (This chapter is specifically concerned with the autonomic system, but it should be remembered that autonomic and endocrine functions are inextricably linked.)

Sympathetic "Local Brains"

During the seventeenth and eighteenth centuries the concept of an involuntary nervous system was developed. It was the anatomical description of chains of ganglia (clusters of nerve cells) lying on either side of the spinal cord, that led to the term "sympathetic nervous system." The ganglia were considered to be "local brains" that kept different parts of the body coordinated and "in sympathy."

It was the French physiologist Claude Bernard (1813–1878) who first proposed that internal regulatory mechanisms were responsible for maintaining a constant internal environment — the

milieu intérieur. Later, in 1900, another French physiologist, Charles Richet, suggested that further refinement of the concept was required when considering the living body. He wrote, "... by apparent contradiction it [the *milieu intérieur*] maintains its stability only if it is excitable and capable of modifying itself according to external stimuli and adjusting in response to stimulation."

It was only during the late nineteenth century that the structure and function of this branch of the nervous system was appreciated fully. The English physiologist J. N. Langley (1852–1925) made some fundamental observations on the autonomic nerves and came to the conclusion that the nerves formed a dual system — the sympathetic branch and the parasympathetic branch. He showed that these two components were both anatomically and functionally distinct. The nerves originated from different parts of the central nervous system, they had reciprocal actions within the body and used different chemicals (neurotransmitters) to transmit

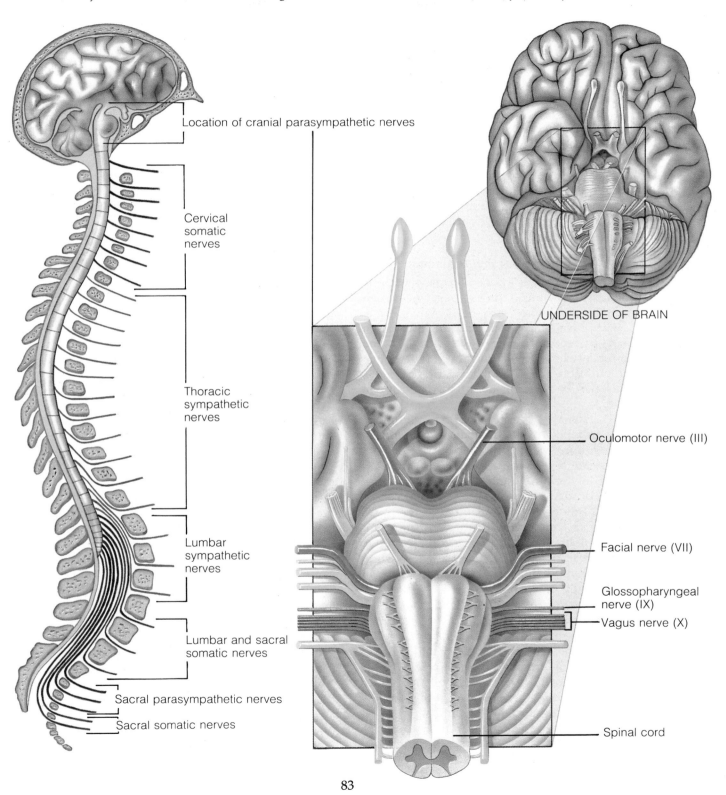

The autonomic nervous system consists of two divisions: the sympathetic and parasympathetic systems. The sympathetic nerves (red) arise from the twelve thoracic (chest) and first three lumbar (lower back) segments of the spinal cord. The parasympathetic nerves (blue) originate from the second, third, and fourth sacral segments (near the base of the spine) and are also distributed through the third, seventh, ninth and tenth cranial nerves (which arise from the underside of the brain and brainstem). The diagram also shows the origins of the other cranial nerves (yellow) and of the somatic nerves (black) from the spinal cord.

Location of cranial parasympathetic nerves

Cervical somatic nerves

Thoracic sympathetic nerves

Lumbar sympathetic nerves

Lumbar and sacral somatic nerves

Sacral parasympathetic nerves

Sacral somatic nerves

UNDERSIDE OF BRAIN

Oculomotor nerve (III)

Facial nerve (VII)

Glossopharyngeal nerve (IX)

Vagus nerve (X)

Spinal cord

83

their electrical signals to the target glands and organs. In fact, it was he who coined the term "autonomic."

In parallel with Langley's work, the American physiologist W. B. Cannon clarified many ambiguities concerning the functions of the autonomic nervous system. He formulated the idea that the sympathetic division was a catabolic (breaking down) and spending system, whereas the parasympathetic component was an anabolic (building up) or conserving system. His belief that the sympathetic nervous system centered around its function during times of emergency led to the original idea of the fight-or-flight reaction, which has endured ever since.

Structure and Functions of the Autonomic System

The autonomic nervous system contrasts with the somatic (voluntary and sensory) nervous system, although some parallels can be drawn between them. Both have simple reflex arcs — information from sensory receptors is transmitted to the spinal cord in sensory (afferent) nerve fibers, and a signal is sent out from the spinal cord in the motor (efferent) nerves to bring about the appropriate response.

Like its somatic counterpart, the autonomic system is arranged in a hierarchical manner. In the central nervous system, more complex reflexes which regulate respiration and blood pressure are integrated in the autonomic center of the lower brainstem, or medulla, whereas those that control the pupils of the eyes are integrated in the upper brainstem, or midbrain (mesencephalon).The highest level of autonomic regulation is found within the rear part of the forebrain, in an area called the hypothalamus. This tiny, complex structure — not much bigger than a soybean — sits at the base of the cerebral hemispheres and regulates autonomic functions such as temperature control and appetite. It also controls many hormone secretions of the endocrine system and receives information from areas of the brain, called the limbic system, which are concerned with emotional and instinctual behavior. Signals from the environment which alter human emotions and behavior are received at the hypothalamus and, in turn, the hypothalamus relays the messages to the brainstem and spinal cord that switch on or off various autonomic responses.

The anatomical arrangement of autonomic nerves emerging from the spinal cord and brainstem differs from that of the skeletal motor nerves of the somatic system. Each motor pathway from the spinal cord comprises only a single motor neuron whose fiber passes out of the cord in a ventral root and along a spinal nerve, directly to a skeletal or striated muscle. Each autonomic pathway, however, comprises two fibers: a preganglionic neuron and a postganglionic neuron. In general, these fibers innervate the smooth muscle of internal organs and tissues.

In the sympathetic branch all the preganglionic neurons are located in the spinal cord and originate from the 12 thoracic and first three lumbar segments of the cord. By contrast, the parasympathetic fibers leave the central nervous system through several of the cranial nerves (III, VII, IX and X) and from the the second, third and fourth sacral segments at the base of the spinal column.

Lying along each side of the spinal cord, from the neck to the hip, there are small "nodules" of nervous tissue, each not much bigger than a match head, and connected to adjacent nodules; these form the sympathetic chains. The nodules are the sympathetic ganglia where insulated (or myelinated) preganglionic fibers connect with the postganglionic neurons. Just after the preganglionic sympathetic nerves emerge from the ventral roots of the spinal cord, they leave the spinal nerves (via the white rami) and dive into one of the ganglia. Here they have three possible pathways: they can connect with the postganglionic neuron in that ganglion, or they can travel up or down the sympathetic chain and connect with a neighbor in another ganglion, or they can pass straight through and connect with outlying ganglia.

All the small uninsulated or unmyelinated fibers that control the caliber of blood vessels, the sweat glands and the tiny muscles (piloerector muscles) that make the hair stand on end, go back into the spinal nerves via the gray rami. Some postganglionic fibers, such as those that go to the heart and lungs, do not rejoin the spinal nerves but go directly to their targets. The postganglionic fibers which regulate the stomach, intestines, liver,

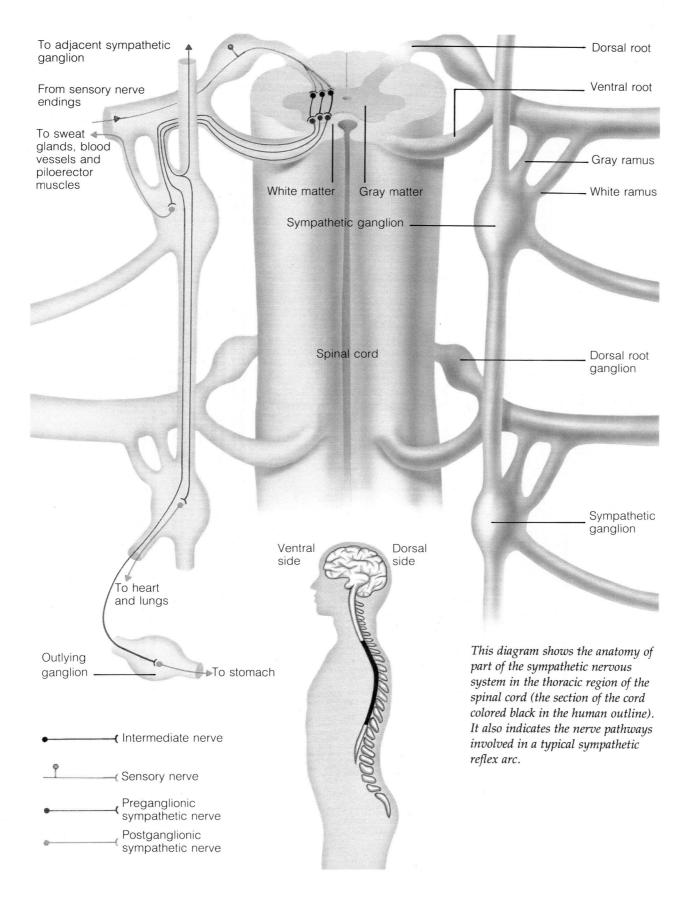

To adjacent sympathetic ganglion

From sensory nerve endings

To sweat glands, blood vessels and piloerector muscles

White matter

Gray matter

Sympathetic ganglion

Spinal cord

To heart and lungs

Outlying ganglion

To stomach

Intermediate nerve

Sensory nerve

Preganglionic sympathetic nerve

Postganglionic sympathetic nerve

Dorsal root

Ventral root

Gray ramus

White ramus

Dorsal root ganglion

Sympathetic ganglion

Ventral side

Dorsal side

This diagram shows the anatomy of part of the sympathetic nervous system in the thoracic region of the spinal cord (the section of the cord colored black in the human outline). It also indicates the nerve pathways involved in a typical sympathetic reflex arc.

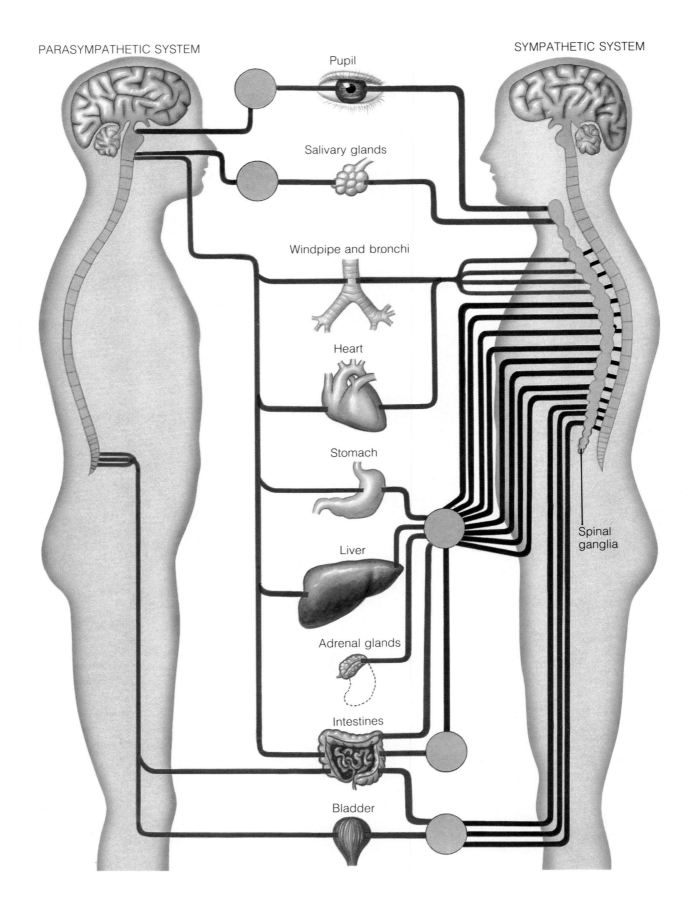

Pupil

Salivary glands

Windpipe and bronchi

Heart

Stomach

Liver

Adrenal glands

Intestines

Bladder

Spinal ganglia

Some of the effects of parasympathetic and sympathetic stimulation are shown opposite. The red pathways indicate that organs are "turned on," blue pathways that they are "turned off." For example, parasympathetic stimulation causes the pupil to contract; saliva production to increase; the windpipe and bronchi to constrict; movements and secretions of the stomach and intestines to increase; and the bladder to contract. It also slows the heart and reduces the liberation of glucose by the liver. Sympathetic stimulation has opposite effects, and causes the adrenal glands to release epinephrine and norepinephrine.

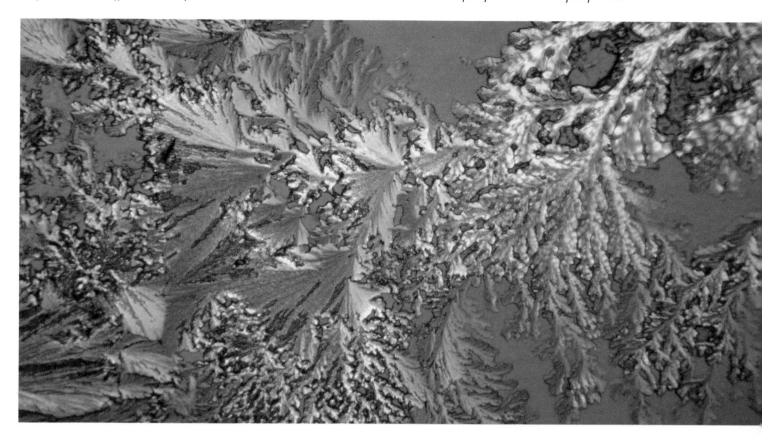

kidneys, bladder and sex organs arise from the outlying celiac and mesenteric ganglia.

There is one sympathetic pathway that does not conform to this general two-neuron arrangement. This is the sympathetic innervation of the two adrenal glands, each of which sits on top of a kidney. In the middle or medullary part of the adrenal gland there are modified postganglionic neurons which do not have axons or fibers projecting to a target organ. Instead, they are crammed full of small secretory granules which release the sympathetic hormones epinephrine and norepinephrine into the bloodstream to stimulate a generalized sympathetic response. The release of these hormones is triggered by preganglionic fibers which pass directly from the spinal cord, through the sympathetic chain, to the adrenal medulla.

The anatomy of the parasympathetic nervous system is different from that of the sympathetic branch. The ganglia do not lie near the spinal cord

Crystals of epinephrine have this multicolored, feathery appearance when illuminated with polarized light and viewed under a microscope (the magnification is about 650 times). Epinephrine is one of the two principal hormones secreted by the adrenal glands in response to stimulation by the sympathetic system; the other is norepinephrine. Together, these two substances produce a generalized "fight-or-flight" sympathetic response.

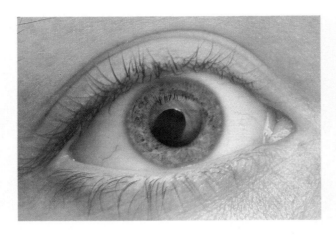

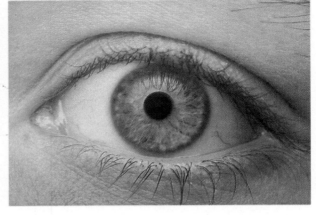

but are instead situated very close to or within the target organs; the preganglionic fibers are relatively long whereas the postganglionic fibers may be a small fraction of an inch in length. Approximately 75 per cent of all the parasympathetic fibers are in the two vagus nerves (Xth cranial nerves) which branch repeatedly, supplying nerves to all the major organs in the chest and abdomen.

The parasympathetic outflow from the other cranial nerves goes to the muscles of the eyes (nerve III), and to the nasal, tear and salivary glands (nerves VII and IX). At the tail end of the spinal cord the remainder of the parasympathetic fibers emerge from three sacral segments and congregate in the pelvic nerves. The branches of these nerves distribute themselves to the intestine, rectum, bladder, the ureters of the kidney and to the external genitalia where they are involved in various sexual responses.

Control of Body Processes

Many organs (for example the eye, the heart, the stomach and parts of the intestine) receive both sympathetic and parasympathetic fibers, and the effects are often reciprocal. But there is no generalization by which it can be predicted whether sympathetic or parasympathetic stimulation will cause excitation or inhibition of a particular organ. For the body as a whole, however, sympathetic stimulation prepares the body for action — by increasing the heart rate and blood pressure, for example — whereas parasympathetic stimulation has the opposite effect.

The amount of light entering the eye is controlled by the autonomic nervous system. In bright light there is a reflex stimulation of the parasympathetic fibers in the third cranial nerve and this constricts the pupil, limiting the amount of light entering the eye. In periods of excitement the sympathetic fibers are stimulated. This dilates the pupils and raises the eyelids, producing the "popeye" effect. Focusing of the lens of the eye is controlled almost exclusively by parasympathetic fibers.

Similarly, the exocrine glands (such as the salivary and sweat glands) are primarily regulated by the parasympathetic system. Parasympathetic fibers cause salivation when the smell of good food reaches the nostrils, and produce copious secretions of digestive juices when we eat a meal. The sympathetic fibers supplying these glands have a reciprocal action, tending to inhibit glandular secretions, and this effect can be felt in the "dry mouth" syndrome associated with stress. In contrast, there is one type of gland which receives only a sympathetic innervation. These are the sweat glands which are stimulated when the temperature of the body rises.

The movement of food out of the stomach and its propulsion along the intestine, by peristalsis, is also assisted by parasympathetic stimulation. Conversely, both motility and secretions of the gastrointestinal tract tend to be inhibited by the sympathetic system. Sympathetics also cause the airways (bronchi) to dilate, thereby facilitating the movement of air into the lungs, whereas the parasympathetic fibers have the opposite effect. In

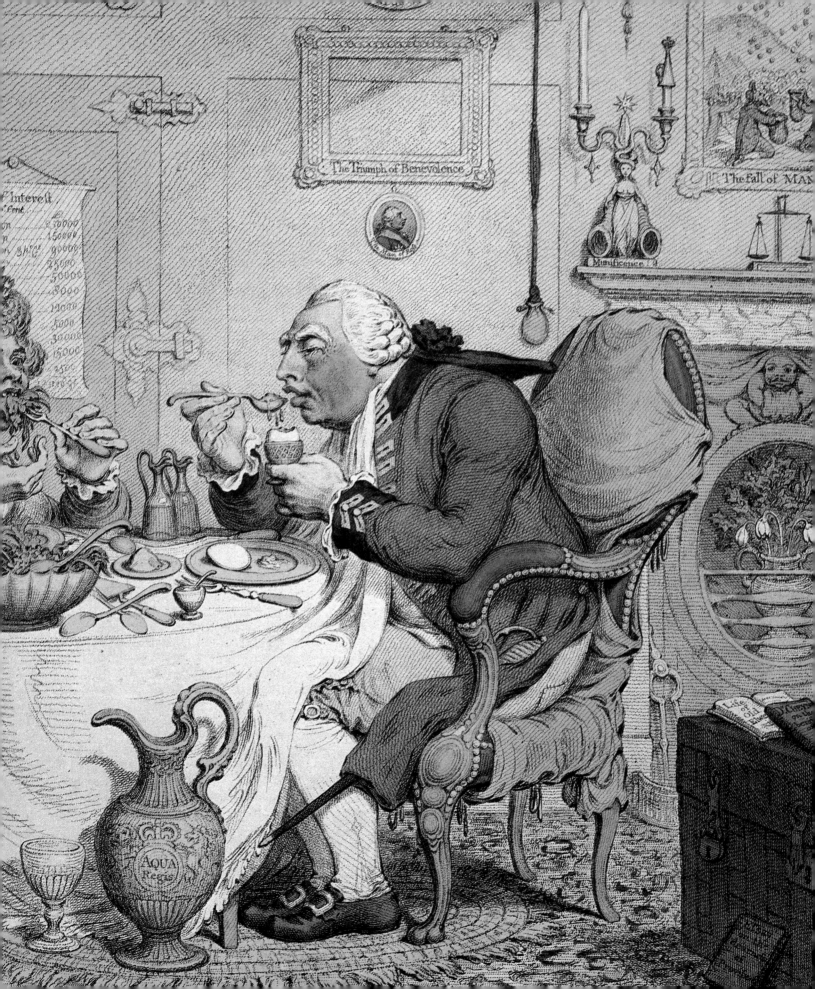

Interest
cent...
70000
150000
90000
25000
5000
8000
10000
5000
3000
1500
250

The Triumph of Benevolence

The Man of...

Munificence

The fall of MAN

AQUA
Regis

fact, a common treatment for asthmatics, who suffer severe constriction of the bronchi, is to inhale a drug which mimics the effects of sympathetic stimulation; the dilated bronchi make breathing easier.

Blood pressure and blood flow are precisely controlled by an extensive autonomic innervation to the heart, arteries and veins. Sympathetic stimulation of cardiac muscle increases the rate of heart beat and the force of the contraction so that more blood is propelled around the body. At the same time, sympathetic stimulation also constricts the smooth muscle fibers surrounding blood vessels, especially those going to the abdomen, and dilates those carrying blood to active skeletal muscles. This directs blood flow to the muscles and away from the digestive tract, which is why exercise soon after a meal may cause stomach cramps. Parasympathetic stimulation slows the heart but has little effect on blood vessels, except those going to the skin of the face. Blushing is due to a huge discharge of parasympathetic neurons.

The autonomic control of heart rate and blood flow is in action continually, regulating minute-to-minute changes in blood pressure. In the main artery coming out of the heart (the aorta), and in the carotid arteries going to the head, there are special stretch receptors referred to as baroreceptors. Essentially these receptors send messages to the autonomic center in the brainstem about the degree of stretch in the arteries. Low blood pressure means there is not much stretch, and so the brainstem sends out messages to increase the rate of heart beat and to restrict the blood flow to the visceral organs until the correct blood pressure is reinstated.

The immediate problem of a severe hemorrhage is a precipitous drop in blood pressure. Due to a reflex sympathetic stimulation by the baroreceptor input, the patient feels cold and looks extremely pale. Very little blood flows to the skin and proportionately more circulating blood is available for the vital organs such as the heart and brain. The opposite effect is seen with high blood pressure. There is more stretch in the arteries and so the baroreceptors reflexly stimulate the vagus nerve to slow down the heart, while sympathetic stimulation dilates some blood vessels and lowers the resistance to blood flow.

There are, of course, many other visceral functions which are under autonomic control. In general these are stimulated by the parasympathetic nerves but inhibited by sympathetic nerves — for example, bile secretion from the gall bladder, urine flow and bladder emptying. Sympathetic stimulation also has metabolic effects and these tend to increase the fuel available for energy. The liver releases stored glucose into the blood circulation, fat stores release fatty acids, and the skeletal muscles break down their own fuel, namely stores of glycogen. Finally, autonomic nerves mediate male and female sexual responses. For example, erection is a parasympathetic response, and ejaculation is a sympathetic response.

The highest level of autonomic control resides in the hypothalamus, where body temperature, hunger and thirst are regulated. The normal human body temperature is approximately 98.6°F and is closely regulated around this set point by means of thermostats or thermoreceptors, which occur both in the skin and within the hypothalamus itself. The skin tends to look flushed when the body temperature rises because the blood vessels in the skin are dilated; more blood flows to the surface and more heat is lost to the environment. At the same time sweating is stimulated by the sympathetic nerves, and heat is lost by evaporation of the sweat.

Conversely, when cold, the body switches on heat-conserving mechanisms and the skin can appear "blue with cold" because all the surface blood vessels are shut down. Shivering begins — involuntary contractions of skeletal muscles which generate heat within the body.

Fever is an interesting adaptation of thermoregulation, because the presence of bacteria or viruses, for example, in some way changes the set point of the hypothalamic thermostat and causes body temperature to rise. A new point, say at 100°F, is set — but the body temperature is still at the old setting of 98.6°F. The patient feels cold, looks pale and shivers until the body temperature reaches 100°F. At the end of a fever, the set point drops back to 98.6°F but the body is still at 100°F. The patient feels hot, looks flushed and sweats until the body temperature is normal again.

The hypothalamic regulation of appetite

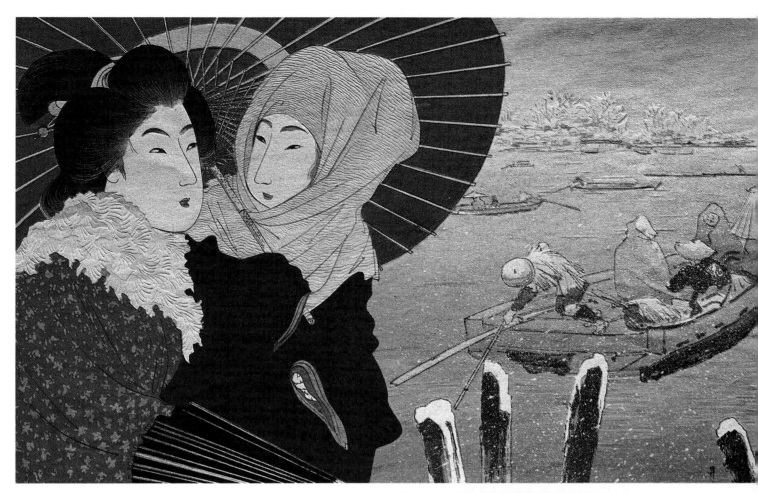

In cold conditions, such as the
winter scene depicted by the Japanese
artist Shoun, the autonomic nervous
system acts to conserve body heat.
One of the mechanisms that achieves
this is a reduction of blood flow to
the surface of the skin by constriction
of the superficial blood vessels. The
effect is vividly illustrated in the
thermograph (right) of a man with
his arms held above his head,
showing the heat generated in the
areas of skin around the armpits.
The colored bars at the bottom
indicate temperature, increasing
sequentially from cool (black) to hot
(white).

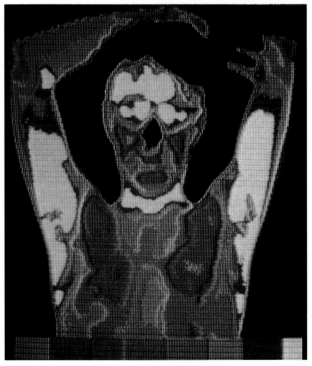

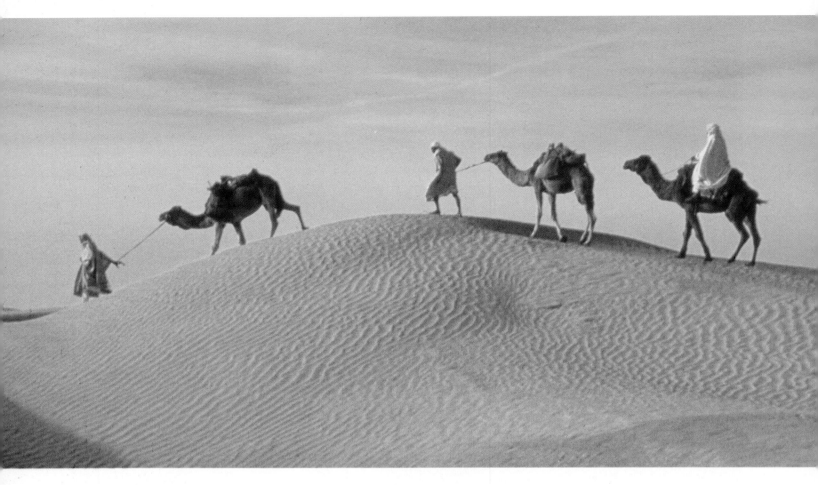

In hot conditions the autonomic nervous system promotes heat loss by initiating mechanisms such as sweating and dilating blood vessels near the surface of the skin. The thermograph (opposite) shows the result of the various heat-loss mechanisms; the colored bars indicate temperature, increasing from black (cool) through white (hot). The coolest areas are the armpits because they are well supplied with sweat glands. Sweating cools the body most effectively in hot, dry conditions — desert climates, for example. In humid conditions sweat evaporates from the body more slowly, reducing and the cooling effect of sweating.

depends upon the interaction of two centers referred to as the "feeding center" and the "satiety center." If the feeding center is destroyed, an animal simply ceases to eat and becomes anorectic. But if the satiety center is destroyed, the animal eats continuously and becomes grossly obese. It seems, therefore, that satiety inhibits the feeding center and helps check the appetite. There appears to be a kind of glucostat function in the satiety center which somehow measures the blood sugar levels and the rate at which glucose is taken up into the nerve cells. When blood sugar is low, less glucose is available for use and the satiety center signals to the feeding center to switch on appetite. A high utilization of glucose and a distended stomach depress appetite via norepinephrine-releasing nerves which run from the brainstem to the hypothalamus.

Also in the hypothalamus there are neurons called osmoreceptors which sense the salt concentration of body fluids, and in this way help to regulate the water content of our bodies by controlling urine flow and the thirst mechanism. An integrated hypothalamic response to a state of

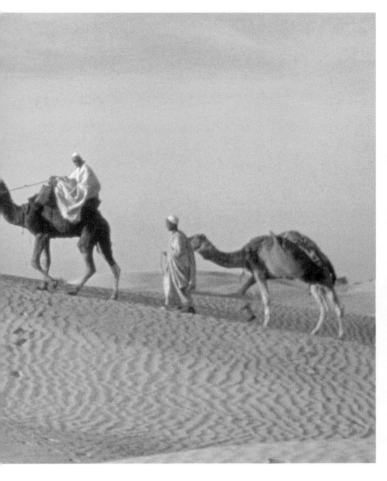

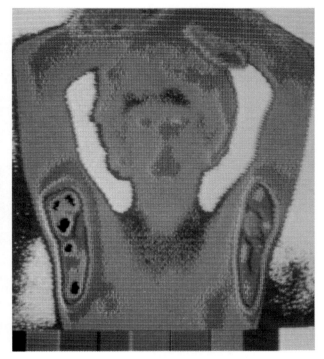

dehydration stimulates water conservation (by inhibiting the volume of urine produced) and at the same time induces a feeling of thirst.

The Chemistry of Autonomic Control

The sympathetic and parasympathetic systems function in unison to coordinate the activities of different parts of the organism. For more than a century it has been known that certain drugs produce effects similar to those produced by stimulating either parasympathetic or sympathetic autonomic nerves. Other preparations appear to have the power to block or reduce the normal effects of stimulating these autonomic nerves.

Chemicals with this type of action are used widely to treat diseases and intensive research to develop more effective drugs continues. What all the drugs have in common is that they either mimic or inhibit the action of acetylcholine or of norepinephrine (noradrenaline). Acetylcholine is used to transmit electrical information from all preganglionic nerve fibers of the autonomic nerves to their respective postganglionic neurons (the same chemical is released from somatic nerves

supplying skeletal muscle). The neurotransmitters released from the postganglionic nerves onto their target cells are different in the two branches of the autonomic system. The parasympathetic postganglionic nerves release acetylcholine, whereas the postganglionic sympathetic nerves generally release norepinephrine (although the sympathetic nerves supplying sweat glands are exceptional, and release acetylcholine). Acetylcholine is therefore the agent responsible for slowing the heart rate and reducing the force of the beat when the vagus nerve is stimulated, and norepinephrine the agent which causes the heart rate to speed up and the beat to become stronger when sympathetic nerves are stimulated.

It is not difficult to make acetylcholine or norepinephrine in a laboratory, and if these synthetic products are injected into the bloodstream and get to their appropriate receptors, they generate responses in an identical manner to their natural counterparts.

The plant kingdom provides a wealth of drugs with an enormous diversity of biological actions, including some that interact with the autonomic

The autonomic nervous system uses several transmitter substances. All preganglionic nerves utilize acetylcholine, but the transmitters released by the postganglionic nerves differ in the sympathetic and

parasympathetic systems. Most sympathetic postganglionic nerves release norepinephrine onto their target effector cells (smooth muscle cells in the intestinal wall, for example), whereas parasympathetic

postganglionic nerves release acetylcholine. In the adrenal glands, however, the secretory cells (which are modified sympathetic postganglionic cells) release norepinephrine and epinephrine.

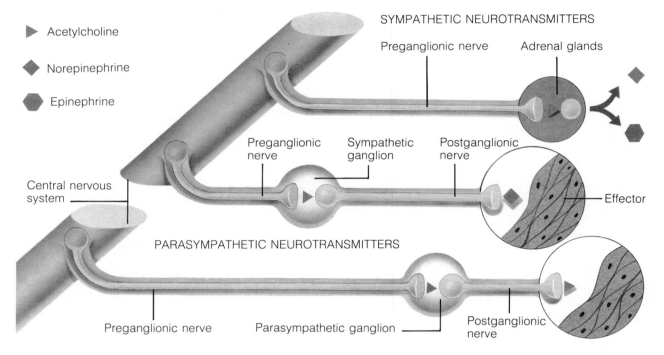

▶ Acetylcholine

◆ Norepinephrine

⬡ Epinephrine

SYMPATHETIC NEUROTRANSMITTERS

Preganglionic nerve   Adrenal glands

Preganglionic nerve   Sympathetic ganglion   Postganglionic nerve

Central nervous system

Effector

PARASYMPATHETIC NEUROTRANSMITTERS

Preganglionic nerve   Parasympathetic ganglion   Postganglionic nerve

nervous system. Nicotine comes from the tobacco plant, and muscarine is a natural product of the toadstool *Amanita muscaria*. The deadly nightshade plant, *Atropa belladonna*, yields a drug (atropine) which has been used for centuries both as a poison and in medicinal and cosmetic preparations. This drug attaches itself to the acetylcholine receptors on the target tissues of the parasympathetic nerves, but has no power to stimulate cells. Atropine prevents communication between parasympathetic nerves and their target cells by denying acetylcholine access to its receptors.

Another plant product, the South American Indian arrow poison curare, has actions similar to that of atropine, except that it exerts its effects only on the nicotine-sensitive acetylcholine receptors. This explains why the most prominent effect of curare is to cause weakness or paralysis of all skeletal muscles.

Both atropine and curare are still used in modern medicine, and their usefulness has increased greatly since effective ways of reversing their paralyzing effects were discovered. One antidote to atropine and curare is also a plant product — physostigmine — obtained from the African

calabar bean. Physostigmine blocks the action of the enzyme cholinesterase, which breaks down and inactivates acetylcholine released from nerve terminals. By so doing, physostigmine prolongs and intensifies the effects of the neurotransmitter, acetylcholine, on the target cells — an effect which is opposite to the effect of either curare or atropine.

Just as there are two types of acetylcholine receptors (sensitive in different ways to nicotine and muscarine), there are also two types of norepinephrine receptors. One, the alpha-type, is involved, for example, in the constriction of blood vessels and the dilator response of the pupil of the eye. On the other hand, speeding of the heart, dilating of the airways (bronchi) and dilation of blood vessels going to the skeletal muscle are responses produced by norepinephrine occupying the so-called beta-type receptors.

Epinephrine, secreted into the circulation from the adrenal medulla, is also able to occupy norepinephrine receptors, and it is through this action that fuel stored in the liver, muscles and fat deposits is released and made available for extra energy requirements.

These two types of receptors can also be selectively blocked by drugs. The natural products of the ergot fungus, which grows on rye, can block the alpha-type norepinephrine receptors, and synthetic drugs have been developed within the last 30 years which selectively antagonize the beta-effects of norepinephrine and epinephrine. These are the so-called "beta blockers" which have a variety of medicinal uses, including the treatment of high blood pressure, abnormal heart rhythms, migraine, and glaucoma (increase of pressure within the eye). Synthetic drugs such as iso-proterenol and salbutamol, which have a norepinephrine-like action and stimulate beta receptors, have also proved useful as medicines, particularly in the treatment of asthma where they are effective in dilating airways in the lung, thus assisting a patient to breathe more easily.

In some types of disease, autonomic neurons fail to exercise proper control over particular bodily functions and drugs are used to restore the equilibrium. Certain people, for example, suffer from abnormally high blood pressure which causes undue strain on the heart and can result in damage to vital organs like the kidney and the retina of the eye. For some reason it seems that the sympathetic nervous system is unable to compensate for the increased blood pressure by widening the diameter of the blood vessels. Fortunately drugs are now available which can make up this deficit.

Voluntary Control of Autonomic Functions

From the base of the spinal cord up to the hypothalamus there is a complex network of outflowing autonomic nerves which continually exert a tonic involuntary control on internal functions. This is achieved by neurotransmitters released from nerve endings, and their recognition by receptors on the target cells. The degree of this "tone" must change in accordance with bodily demands, and so an equally complex system of sensory (afferent) nerves from the internal visceral organs sends information to the autonomic integrating centers. Sometimes this information from the visceral receptors reaches consciousness and in response a certain degree of conscious control can be exerted over some autonomic functions. For example, stretch receptors in the

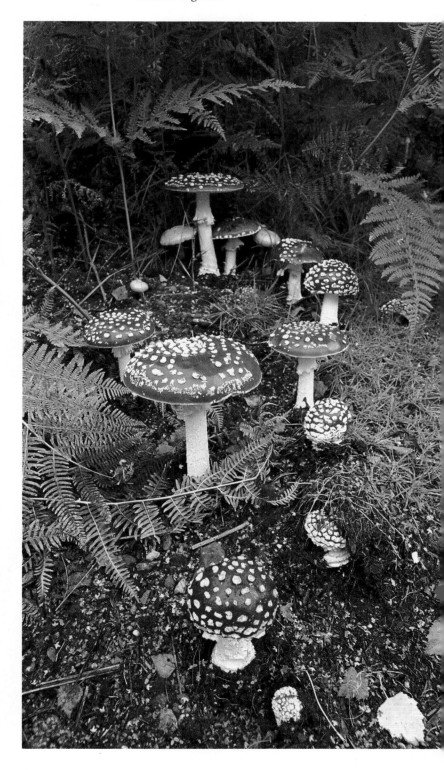

95

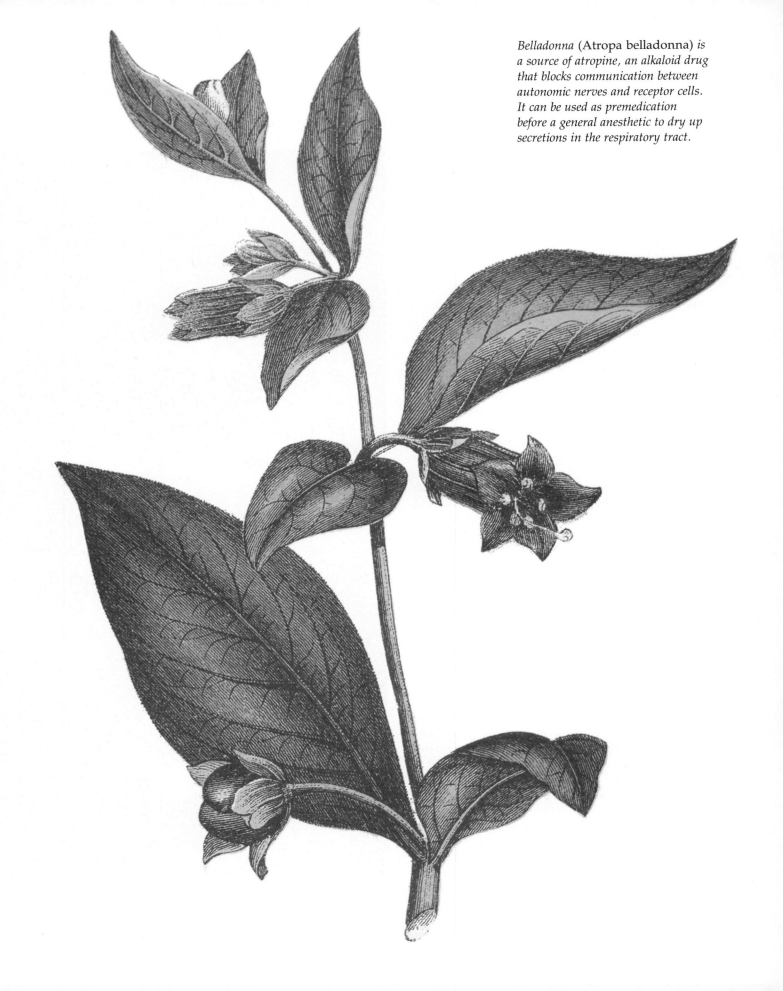

Belladonna (Atropa belladonna) *is a source of atropine, an alkaloid drug that blocks communication between autonomic nerves and receptor cells. It can be used as premedication before a general anesthetic to dry up secretions in the respiratory tract.*

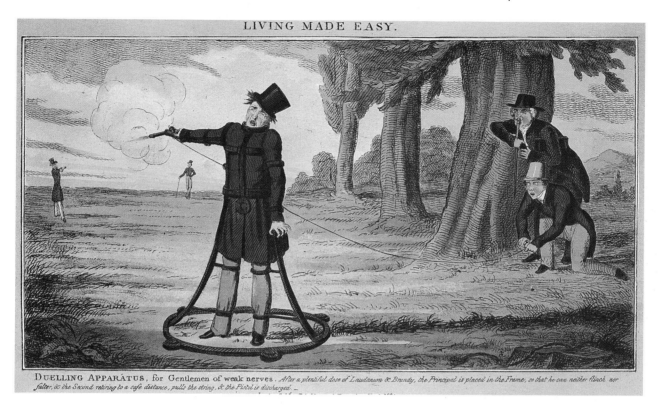

LIVING MADE EASY.

DUELLING APPARATUS, for Gentlemen of weak nerves. *After a plentiful dose of Laudanum & Brandy, the Principal is placed in the Frame, so that he can neither flinch nor falter, & the Second retiring to a safe distance, pulls the string, & the Pistol is discharged.—*

wall of the bladder signal when it is full, but we can consciously inhibit the parasympathetic reflex of bladder emptying.

By contrast, perturbations in the external environment, perceived through the sense organs, can stimulate involuntary responses of the autonomic system. The best example of this is the fight-or-flight response. As a way of summarizing the general effects of the autonomic nervous system, this response now needs consideration in more detail.

Imagine that your wallet has just been snatched and the thief is running down the street. You are angry and distressed and your hypothalamus responds. Immediately the stimulated sympathetic system releases norepinephrine from nerve terminals and the adrenal medulla secretes epinephrine and norepinephrine into the bloodstream. The heart rate increases, blood pressure rises, hairs stand on end, and blood flow to the internal organs such as the intestines declines. The spleen (a blood reservoir) contracts and expels extra blood into the circulation, while the vessels supplying the skeletal muscles dilate. You shout for help and begin running after the thief. Fuel is needed for the pursuit so the alerted sympathetic system stimulates the release of stored glucose from the liver, and the conversion of muscle glycogen to glucose. But the fuel must be burned to release energy for running and so the airway passages dilate and more oxygen gets into the lungs; the pupils dilate for more acute vision.

You are running as fast as you can. Exercise produces internal heat and body temperature rises; you begin to sweat. Meanwhile the parasympathetic system has been switched off, your mouth is dry and digestion stops. In one massive autonomic response your body has involuntarily channeled all your regulatory functions into the act of pursuit. You have the best chance your body can give you.

And that chance has been given to you courtesy not only of the autonomic system but also of the endocrine secretions of hormones, both functions working in unison and inextricably linked.

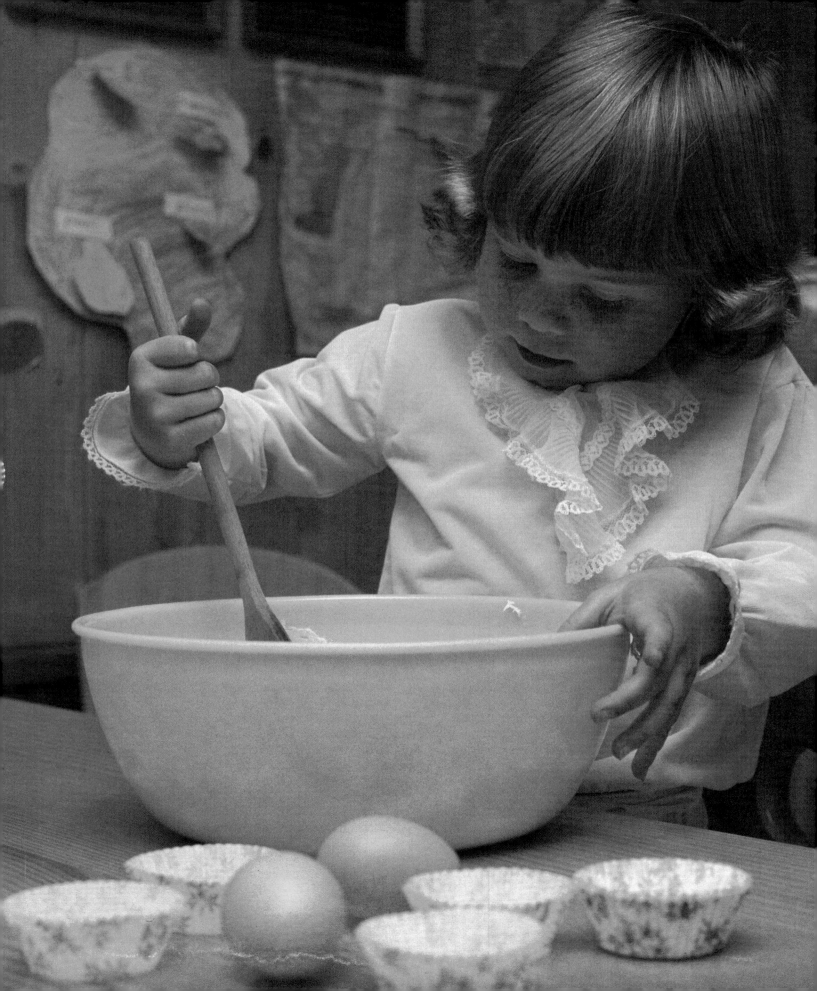

Chapter 6

Conception to Completion

Each human being begins life as a combination of two cells, a female ovum and a much smaller male sperm. This tiny unit, no bigger than a period on this page, contains all the information needed to enable it to grow into the complex structure of the human body. The mother has only to provide nutrition and protection.

It takes forty weeks for a baby to develop inside the protection of the womb. The nervous system itself starts to develop as early as the beginning of the third week and is the first major structure to become visible from the mass of cells which make up the embryo. Scientists have studied its development in microscopic detail, and although there are still some mysteries to unravel, many of the developmental disorders of the nervous system are now understood.

The First Days of Life

Three to four days after the ovum has been fertilized, a small ball of cells begins to travel down the Fallopian tube towards the womb. This ball is the morula and is formed as the original cell divides again and again. By the end of the first week the morula implants into the soft wall of the uterus. If the ball were sliced in half at this point, two chambers would be visible inside, squashed together like a pair of bubbles. The cells squashed between the chambers are called the embryonic disk and these cells form most of the body's tissues. The cells on one side are destined to become the skin and nervous system, and those on the other side will eventually become the lining of the gut.

The embryonic disk lengthens slightly as the days pass, and by day 18 from fertilization the first signs of the nervous system appear. A day later a groove forms, like the midline of a date pit. The groove becomes increasingly deep, and its two long edges fold toward each other, eventually touching first in the middle, then closing to form a cylinder open at each end. The cylinder is known as the

The rapidity with which the nervous system of a young child develops from birth enables most children to have a high degree of control of their movements by the age of two years. Even so, manipulation of tools and neuromuscular coordination are not perfect at that stage and continue to improve through learning processes and with age.

After fertilization an egg undergoes rapid cleavage and forms the embryonic disk at about two weeks. The brain and spinal cord evolve from a region of this disk, known as the primitive groove, which is visible

at 16 days. It thickens and gives rise to the neural plate (the first sign of the central nervous system), at about 18 days. The sides of the neural groove rise and start to fold in so that at about 22 days they meet to

form the neural tube. The newly-formed tube is surrounded only by wedge-shaped neuroepithelial cells. These cells divide to produce neuroblasts, which comprise the mantle layer and are the future gray

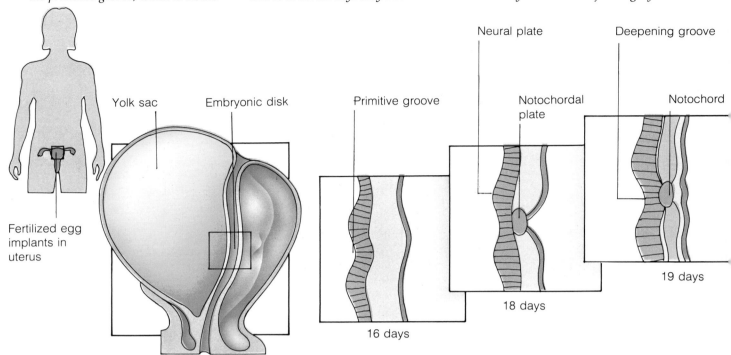

Fertilized egg implants in uterus

Yolk sac

Embryonic disk

Primitive groove

Neural plate

Notochordal plate

Deepening groove

Notochord

16 days

18 days

19 days

neural tube and on each side of it another important structure is forming called the neural crest. This grows up around the neural tube until it encloses it.

While all this is happening segments appear at regular intervals along the embryo. These are called somites and turn into other organs as the embryo grows. The embryo at four-and-a-half weeks old measures only one-fifth of an inch, but it is already attached by the beginnings of the umbilical cord which holds it suspended from the uterine wall in the protective amniotic fluid.

In an adult the bones of the back, or vertebrae, have corresponding muscles (myotomes) and skin structures (dermatomes) supplied by a pair of spinal nerves; it is from the somites on the embryo that these structures form.

The Spinal Cord Develops

If it were possible to look into the amniotic sac at this stage we would see a blob of cells stuck on the end of a stalk. It does not look at all human. In fact, it is unrecognizable as any form of animal, and appears more like a soft chrysalis. Gradually, though, one end of the chrysalis enlarges into three

swellings. This is the beginning of the brain. A cavity within the three swellings spreads down into the developing spinal cord and is to be maintained throughout life, representing the communicating chambers through which fluid washes from the brain through to the spinal cord.

The spinal cord now consists of three layers arranged around a central tube, and within it the primitive nerve cells, or neuroblasts, are beginning to grow. The "factory" that produces them is a tissue known as the neuroepithelium. As the numbers of neuroblasts increase, the cord gradually changes shape; areas at the front and back both enlarge to form the characteristic cross-sectional butterfly-wing shape of the adult cord, with a deep groove on the front (ventral) surface.

The central nervous system is made up of two principal cell types: the neurons, which are the cells that conduct the impulses, and the glial cells which hold everything together. One interesting thing about neurons is that once they have formed they lose their ability to divide and reproduce themselves. They can alter their shape, size and functions — that is to say, they can differentiate —

matter of the spinal cord. The neuroblasts become neurons and develop fibers which extend outward. The axons of the fibers make up the marginal layer of the spinal cord and become myelinated, when they form

the white matter of the cord. The neural tube (called the central canal by 30 days) is divided by longitudinal and lateral grooves which give the cord its characteristic butterfly shape by about 35 days of

the embryo's life. At the age of four weeks (bottom) an embryo's nervous system comprises the brain, neural tube and spinal cord. The brain at this stage makes up one-third of the embryo's size.

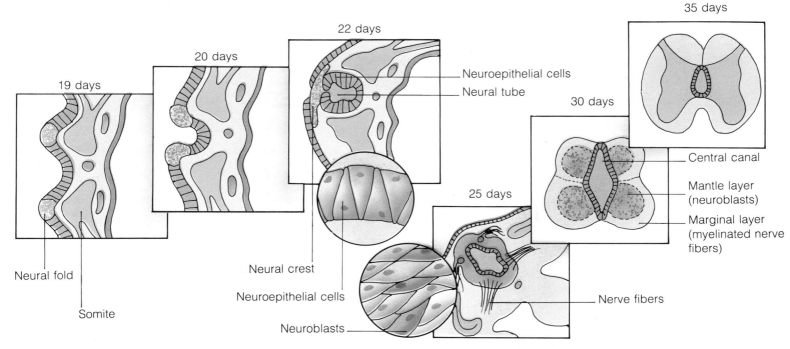

19 days

Neural fold

Somite

20 days

22 days

Neuroepithelial cells

Neural tube

Neural crest

Neuroepithelial cells

Neuroblasts

25 days

30 days

35 days

Central canal

Mantle layer (neuroblasts)

Marginal layer (myelinated nerve fibers)

Nerve fibers

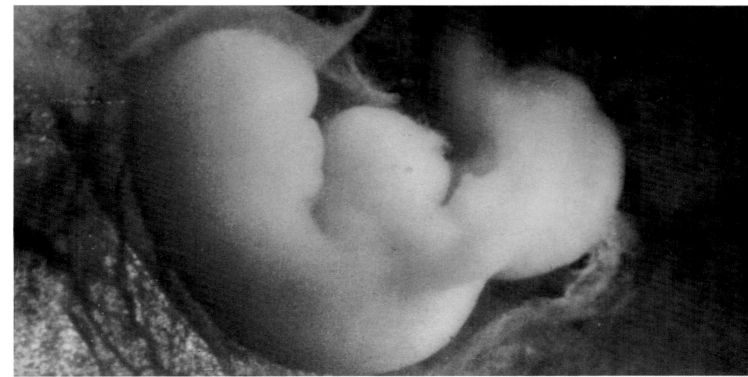

101

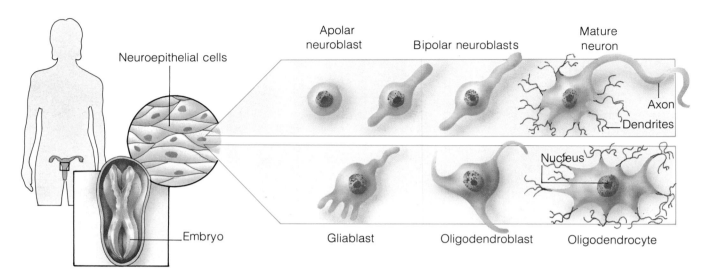

but once formed, they never increase their number.

So how does a neuroblast become a nerve cell? Initially the neuroblast is a round cell, but soon two "limbs" stretch out; one limb becomes longer and the other develops a mass of smaller branches. Meanwhile, the neuroepithelial factory cells inside the spinal cord concentrate on producing neuroblasts. Once the correct number has been made, the factory starts instead to turn out glial cells which make up the supporting structure of the central nervous system. When this task is completed the factory changes its output yet again and makes cells this time of a type to line the inside of the spinal cord itself.

At this stage the embryo looks a bit like a hot dog in a bun. The hot dog is the neural tube housing the neuroepithelial cells and the bun is the neural crest. The neural crest is also a factory for the production of cells, but it has a much more severe task than the other factory. It makes cells not only for nerve fiber coverings (Schwann cells) and the meninges that surround the brain and spinal column, but also cells for teeth (odontoblasts), cells to give the skin its color (melanocytes), and cells for part of the adrenal glands (chromaffin cells). Scientists are still trying to unravel the mystery of the force that guides the cells to create the parts of the body far away from the spinal cord and brain.

At this point it is worthwhile to look again at the classic anatomy of an adult spinal nerve as it leaves the spinal cord. The cell bodies of the motor root lie in the spinal cord itself, whereas the cell bodies of the sensory root are housed outside the spinal cord in the dorsal root ganglion. The reason for this can now be explained. Motor nerve cells are made by the neuroepithelial factory which is housed in the neural tube (the beginnings of the spinal cord) and the sensory nerve cells are made in the neural crest cell factory which lies outside the beginnings of the spinal cord.

Most axons in the nervous system are surrounded by a myelin sheath which acts like the insulation on an electric cord. The myelin sheath is made of Schwann cells whose nuclei lie close to the axon as their cytoplasm containing the fatlike myelin wraps round the axon like paper tightly wrapped around a pencil. The Schwann cells are made in the neural crest cell factory and are then "exported" along the long arms (axons) of the nerve cells which they eventually envelop. Many Schwann cells are needed to surround an axon — one cell with its wraparound sheath takes up approximately one twenty-fifth of an inch on the axon, which looks white because of the covering of myelin. Some axons, especially those in the autonomic nervous system, are never myelinated. Alternatively, the myelin sheath can wrap around more than one axon at a time, and may enclose as many as 20 axons. The nerve fibers in the spinal cord are also covered in myelin, but this insulation

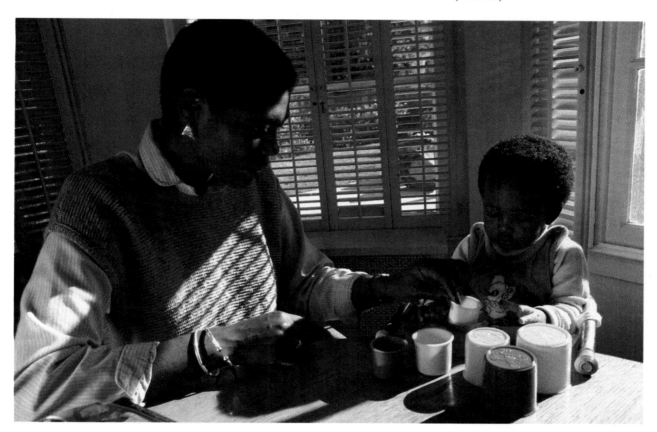

is made from glial cells, not from Schwann cells.

Myelination of nerve cells take many months to complete. It is the second year of life following birth before the task is finished — just in time to coincide roughly with a baby's development of more refined limb movements.

A Human Form Takes Shape

About four-and-a-half weeks after fertilization the embryo's arms and legs begin to appear. The surface of the embryo thickens and small "buds" then come out on either side. At first the buds look round, but soon they flatten out into small paddles. Over the next four weeks an amazing change occurs. These blobs of tissue grow continuously outwards from the body until, by eight weeks, the embryo has arms and legs, fingers and toes. By now it is recognizably human and eyes and ears can be clearly discerned.

As the limb buds grow, so they pull with them

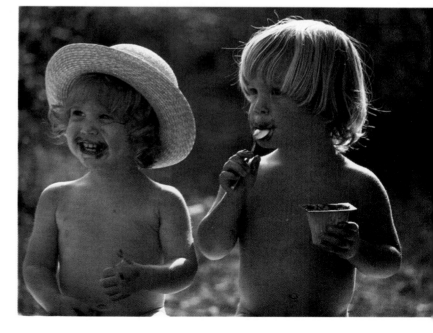

The development of the fetus and the position of the placenta are recorded by inaudible, very high frequency sound (ultrasound) which is passed through the mother's abdomen and does not harm her or the fetus.

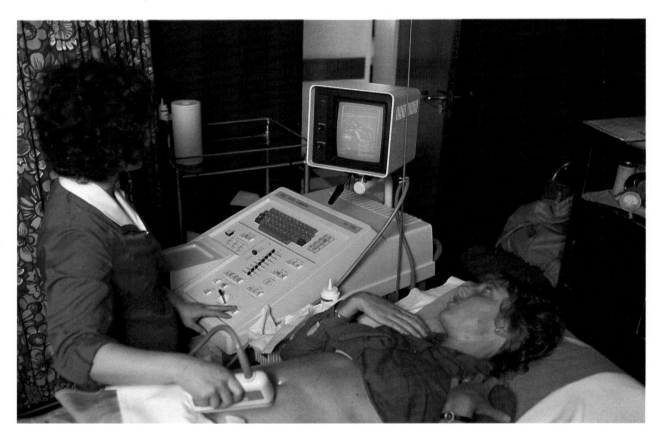

somites that form the dermatomes of the skin and myotomes of the muscles in the embryo's arms. The leg buds develop in the same way. Moreover, as the somites grow and lengthen they take with them their segmental nerves. The peripheral nervous system is thus pulled out along the limbs to all the outlying extremities.

By the time the fetus is three months old it looks like a tiny baby, with miniature features accurate in every detail. Within the body major changes are underway. The neural tube no longer exists; instead, the fetus has a backbone with spinal nerves coming out at right angles all the way down its length. During the next few months the backbone grows faster than the spinal cord, so that the spinal nerves have to travel down inside the vertebral canal to reach the hole through which they are to exit. By the end of the fifth month the spinal cord has lengthened and thickened, but the end of the spinal cord — which once reached the coccyx — is

at the level of the upper sacrum. This process continues, and by birth the difference in length between the spinal cord and the backbone is such that the cord's lower end is at the level of the third lumbar vertebra.

And the discrepancy does not stop there. After birth, the spinal column continues to outstrip the cord, so that in a fully-grown adult, the spinal cord reaches the lower border of the first lumbar vertebra. To adjust to this difference of length, the spinal nerves have to grow longer in order to reach their own exit hole.

The changing difference in length between the bony canal and the cord inside is important in connection with some childhood disorders of the spinal cord. If the nerves are caught in the canal, for example, problems in the legs might well appear as the child grows and the tension on the nerves gradually increases.

Physicians use this length difference to the

patient's advantage in many ways. If, for instance, it is necessary to draw off a sample of the fluid that washes around the spinal cord, a needle can be inserted into the lower lumbar region where the possibility of damage to the cord is avoided because the descending spinal nerves at that level have relatively more room. The sample of cerebrospinal fluid drawn by this lumbar puncture process can then be sent to the laboratory for analysis.

Development of the Autonomic Nervous System

In order to trace the development of the part of the nervous system that controls our automatic responses, such as sweating, heartbeat and the movement of the bowels, it is necessary to return to the five-week-old embryo. The system, known as the autonomic nervous system, is divided into two parts: the sympathetic and parasympathetic nervous systems. The two are in competition with each other in such a way that, for example, the sympathetic nervous system increases the heart rate, but the parasympathetic nervous system decreases it.

Neuroblasts destined to form the sympathetic nervous system are manufactured in the neural crest factory. From here they travel around each side of the embryo's spinal cord to lie alongside the main blood vessel that runs through the embryo. The neuroblasts line up along a nerve fiber and look like a string of beads. The beads are made of groups of cells and are called the sympathetic ganglia. The complete string is known as the sympathetic chain and there is a chain on each side of the large blood vessel, the dorsal aorta.

Some sympathetic neuroblasts are made in the neural crest factory, but instead of joining the chain they are "exported" to more distant locations where they gather together to form other ganglia. The solar plexus, for example, is an autonomic ganglion which lies over the blood vessels for the bowels. Long arms (axons) stretch out from each ganglion to feed nerve impulses to the bowels.

Often long axons do not leave the ganglion directly. In the sympathetic chain an axon may travel up and down the chain before leaving it. The fibers leaving a ganglion have no white myelin insulation on them, and are therefore called a gray communicating ramus.

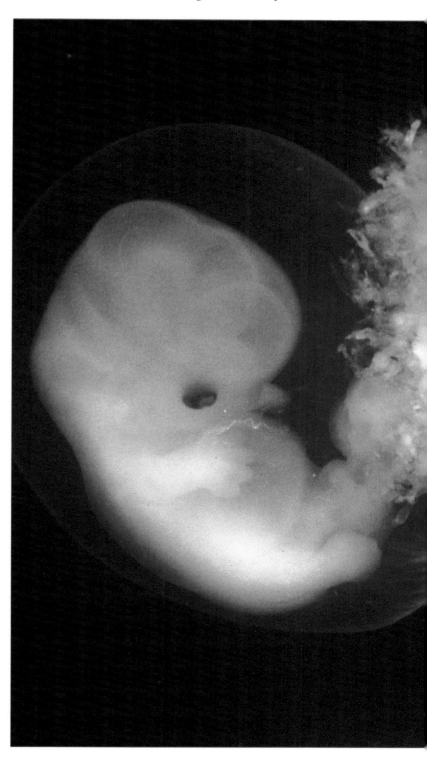

The spiral ganglion in the organ of Corti in the ear develops in the third month of an embryo's life. It receives impulses and sends them to the brain through the auditory fibers of the eighth cranial nerve.

By means of trick photography a composite image can be constructed which conveys the idea of the nervous system in a child as analogous to the electrical wiring and circuitry of a machine.

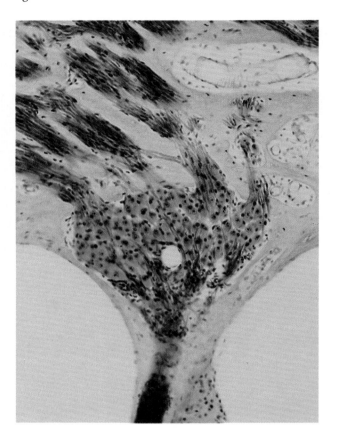

The neural crest factory also "exports" cells to glands which lie just above each kidney, called the adrenal glands. The cells congregate in the middle of these glands and produce the hormone epinephrine (adrenalin) which has the same effect on the body as the sympathetic nervous system.

To get an overall picture of the sympathetic nervous system, imagine the outlying ganglia as telephone extensions in an office. It has been seen how they connect with other extensions along their nerve fibers, but how do they connect with the national telephone network, in this case the central nervous system? The connections form from fibers which grow out from the spinal cord after being manufactured by the neuroepithelial factory. They grow into the ventral root which is already there, join up with the dorsal root fibers coming from behind, and run along side by side in the spinal nerve. Where the spinal nerve goes past the sympathetic chain, sensory fibers form a connec-

tion known as a synapse with the sympathetic nerve cells, and the telephone system becomes fully operational.

The cells for the parasympathetic nervous system are manufactured in the other factory, the neuroepithelium. (It was this factory which made the connecting fibers that grew out toward the sympathetic nervous system.) From here, parasympathetic neurons are "exported" to four of the twelve cranial nerves; unlike the sympathetic ganglia they tend to group together and form ganglia at the same level as the organ they effect, so their fibers are very short. Target organs include the muscles of the pupil of the eye, the tear and salivary glands, and many areas of the bowel.

The Beginnings of the Brain

It is the relative size and capacity of the human brain that sets humankind apart from other animals. Although it is possible to watch it grow from a tiny mass of cells into a complex organ capable of original thought, the brain withholds a myriad secrets.

Imagine again the embryo on day 25, a tiny curled shape around a "stick". The neural tube is closed, and at the head end are three swellings. The one nearest the spinal cord is the hindbrain (rhombencephalon), the next is the midbrain (mesencephalon), and the one at the top is the forebrain (prosencephalon). At this stage the bulges are all of roughly the same size; later one area of the brain outgrows the rest.

As the months pass, the original hindbrain gives rise to two important structures, the cerebellum and the pons. The cerebellum controls balance and coordination during life, and the pons (which means "bridge") becomes a major crossroads at the base of the brain through which many fibers to and from the spinal cord pass. The midbrain forms the upper brainstem, which is principally a pathway to and from the cerebral hemispheres and the nuclei of the forebrain.

The forebrain soon outstrips the other areas in size. Within it grows the thalamus, for receiving and relaying messages, and the hypothalamus, which is the regulation center for — among other things — the emotions.

By 13 weeks the forebrain has grown into two

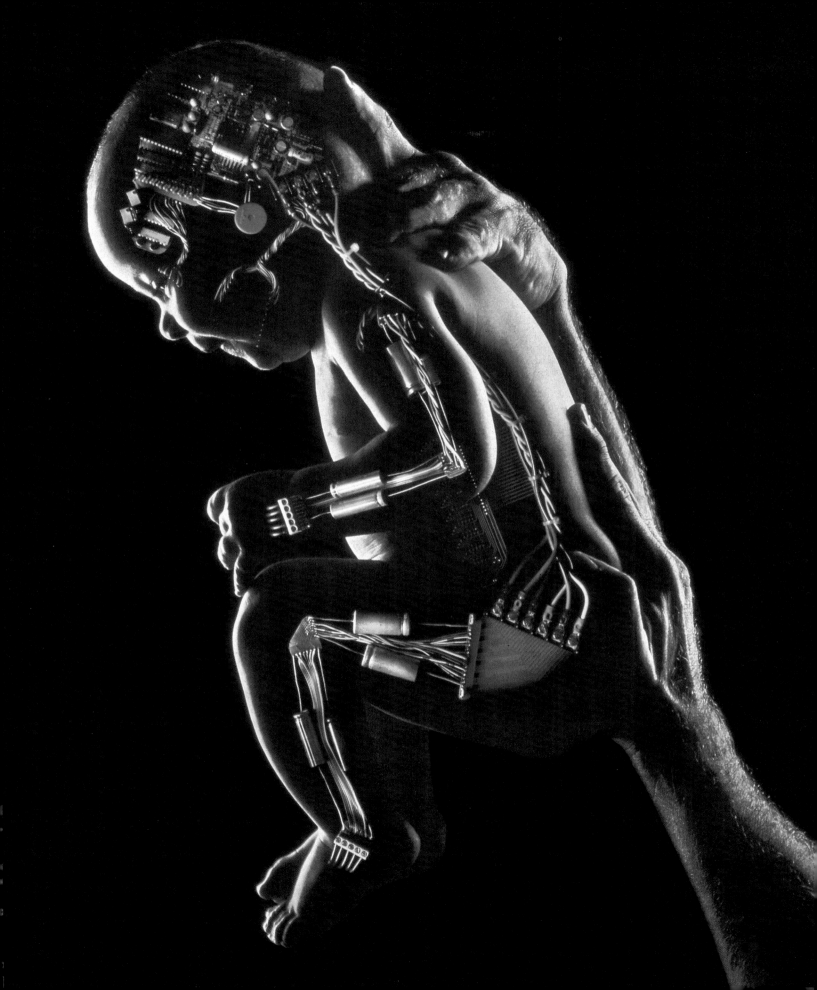

The fissured, contorted mass that is the human brain starts off as a smooth cerebral hemisphere and gradually develops its convoluted form as the fetus approaches maturity.

A baby surrounded by activity develops its nervous system quicker than one in a relatively dull environment because greater stimulation increases the myelination of the nerve fibers.

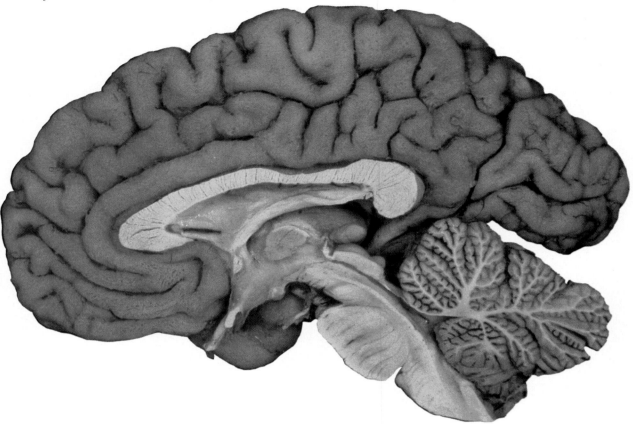

huge cerebral hemispheres with smooth surfaces. But as these continue to grow within the confined space of the skull, their surface is crumpled into gyri (hills) and sulci (valleys), which vastly increase the surface area. It is from the forebrain that the personality of the cerebral hemispheres emerges, that intellect develops, and that original thought may be expressed.

The pituitary gland housed beneath the hemispheres has vital responsibilities throughout life. It produces hormones that control other hormone-producing glands, and regulates the rate at which the body grows. It is directly controlled by the brain, from which part of it develops; the other part comes from the primitive mouth.

At three weeks, a pouch forms in the roof of the embryo's primitive oral cavity, and grows upwards to be cut off from the mouth by week eight. It joins up with a bud growing down from the forebrain, and the two together form the pituitary gland.

From Birth and Onward

A child is born. He or she is able to survive outside the protection of the mother's womb, to breathe, feed and cry for attention. But the nervous system has not yet completed its development. The cerebral hemispheres of the brain still have a great deal of growing to do, and many of the fibers along which the impulses run are not yet fully myelinated. This does not mean that fibers cannot conduct the impulses without the myelin insulation, but that the rate of conduction is considerably slower.

The baby's motor and sensory abilities increase day by day, and the skills he or she acquires roughly coincide with the myelination of the fibers conducting those particular impulses. An interesting thing is that the myelination is not responsible for any increase in a skill. On the contrary; there is now strong evidence to show that the more a nerve fiber is stimulated (that is, the more a skill is actively

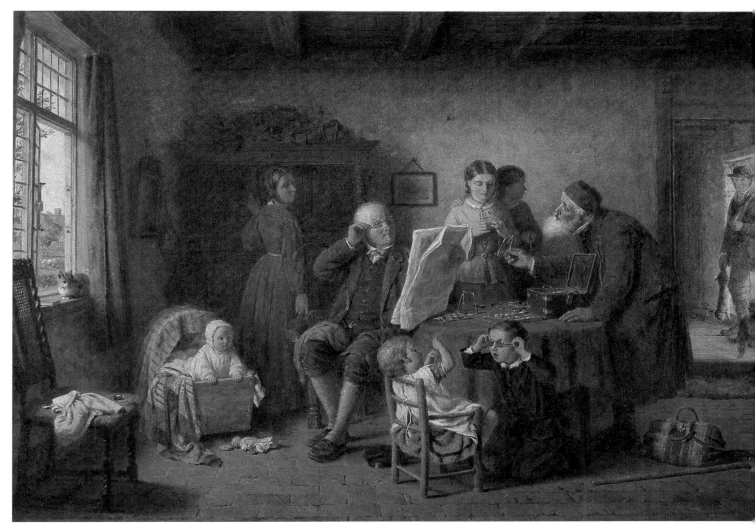

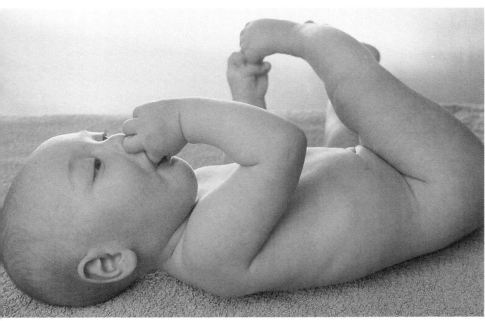

Soon after birth a child has control over little of its body, and its movements are dictated by reflexes. Its fingers grip around any object such as its toes or the fingers held out to it by another person.

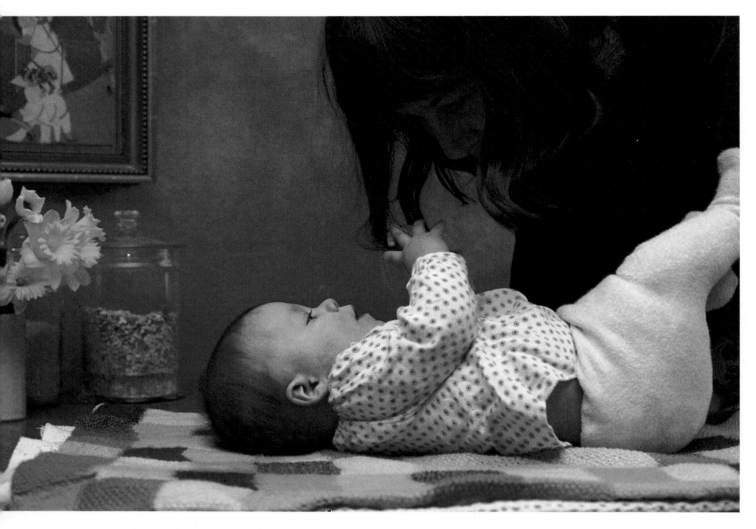

At the age of about six months a baby's optic nerves are myelinated; the baby can see objects clearly enough to lean forward and touch them, and to be able to recognize close members of the family.

used), the quicker the rate of myelination. So the baby surrounded by interesting sights and sounds does indeed develop a mature nervous system more quickly than the child who lies looking at a blank ceiling all day.

At birth the baby — say he's a boy — is a victim of his own muscular activity. A sudden noise makes him jump with every limb and fiber of his being; he expresses hunger or pain by writhing his whole body, and he seems to be in control of nothing. The inhibitory role of the brain has not yet come into play and the baby lives by reflexes. A touch on his cheek makes him turn his head and open his mouth in expectation of food. He has a sucking reflex, his fingers grip around any object placed on his palm, and his feet step out if he is held so that they lightly touch the floor.

One of the most bizarre reflexes at this age is the swimming reflex. If the newborn baby is submerged in water, his face downward, he automatically holds his breath and his arms and legs rhythmically flick him forward in the water. But past the age of four months, water produces fear in a baby, his movements are uncoordinated, and he inhales and swallows water.

These reflexes are with us throughout our lives, but as the brain develops it overrides them. Tragically, they can reemerge if disease causes the brain to deteriorate. An elderly person can regain a rooting reflex when touched on the cheek and a grasp reflex when touched on the palm. This is indeed Shakespeare's "second childishness."

By the age of three months the baby has his body more under control. He breathes steadily, he can control his body temperature, and he responds to the things he sees. The optic nerves are well myelinated by now: if a toy is held out to him he strains his body forward and expresses excitement by waving his arms and legs. He is making early voluntary responses.

By six months the tracts of the spinal cord are well myelinated at shoulder level and it is possible to see that the baby now has good control of his upper body and limbs, but that his legs are not at the same stage of motor control. He can now reach out and take a toy when it is offered, he can even pick it up when he drops it. He recognizes his close family as different from strangers. In the baby's brain the surface area of the cerebral hemisphere is still increasing and the baby has some control over his own destiny. By nine months he is a skillful crawler, in control of his voluntary actions and curious to investigate every inch of the limited world around him. A few months later he is testing his feet and legs, stimulating the fibers in readiness for walking. He holds on to the edge of a table and pulls himself to a standing position, jiggles up and down on the spot, and moves sideways holding the table. Throughout his development the baby exercises the skills he needs long before he ever uses them.

By 12 months of age the different areas of a baby's brain are of the same proportions as an adult brain, although smaller. The baby is on the threshold of an important landmark in development: he is about to walk on two feet and develop a language he can use for communication. The emotions he shows are many — anger, fear, jealousy, happiness, and even sympathy — and whereas in adult life

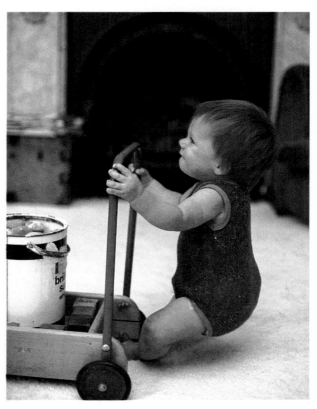

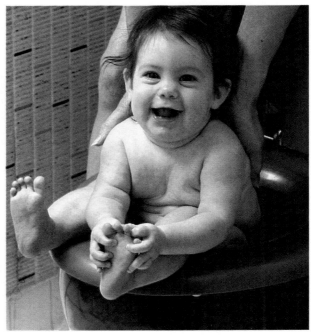

111

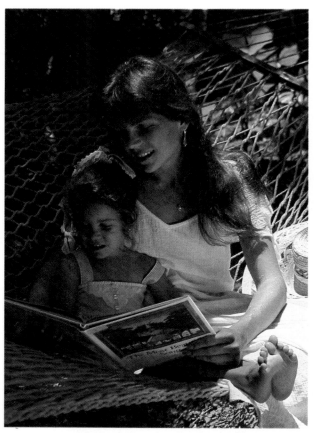

A child's mental processes have advanced, at two years of age, to the point where concentration on an activity is possible for several minutes, whether in reading or playing.

outward displays of many of these emotions are voluntarily controlled, the one-year-old's facial expressions portray every feeling without censure.

By the time a child is two years old, all the structures of the spinal cord, brainstem and cerebellum are myelinated. He can run, his balance is generally good, and he can carry out some simple tasks without looking at his hands. He has a good idea of where he is in the space around him. When he speaks he uses simple sentences. And he has or is soon to have control over his bladder and bowels, which is a sign of advanced activity in the frontal cortex of the brain.

By the age of two, mental processes are quite advanced. He wants to learn, he asks questions, he can solve a simple problem by referring back to his memory of an experience. He can concentrate longer, and may look at a book on his own for nearly six minutes. He has a personality, and although it is not fully developed it is definitely different from those of his siblings.

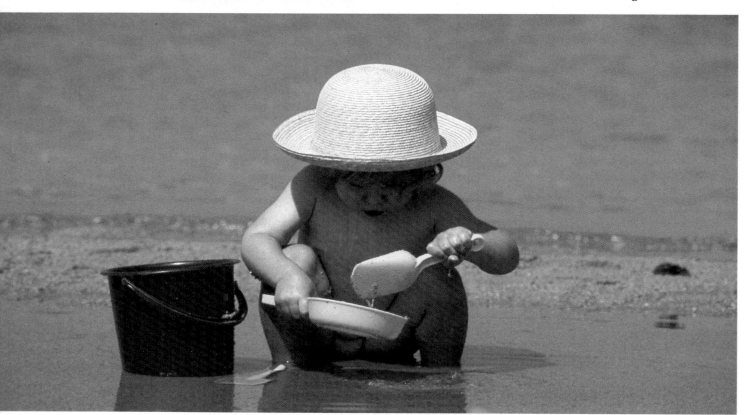

This, then, is really the end of babyhood, and although the nervous system continues to grow (as does the rest of the body), it is not developing in the true sense of the word. The child instead adapts, modifies and perfects the wealth of skills learned during the previous two years.

Development at Risk

If an embryo is not developing properly it usually aborts. This automatic rejection probably accounts for most of the 60 per cent of pregnancies that miscarry. Occasionally, however, a damaged or imperfect fetus grows to term and the abnormality appears as a congenital malformation.

One of the most common congenital malformations of the nervous system, spina bifida, occurs when the neural tube does not close completely. The defect varies in severity: the mildest form, spina bifida occulta, occurs when the bones of the lower back fail to make a complete circle around the spinal cord. The gap may be no more than a hairline crack. The skin over it is normal, although there may be a tuft of hair or birthmark in the middle of the back. The condition may be undetected (occult) throughout life because it never causes any problems. If the defect is wide, however, nerve tissue pushes up under the skin and a swelling is visible at birth. The membrane overlying the protruding nerves or spinal cord is very fragile and easily damaged.

Surgical techniques to deal with the more serious forms of spina bifida are being refined all the time. Many cases can now be repaired at birth even though the child may not gain full control of the legs, bladder or bowels.

Hydrocephaly is a developmental abnormality in which cerebrospinal fluid is prevented from escaping from the chambers of the brain known as the ventricles. Fluid accumulates under pressure, making the brain and head larger than normal. It is now possible to put a tube into the ventricles to drain the fluid into the body cavity where it is quickly absorbed.

Why these abnormalities occur is not yet known with certainty, but we do know that they happen at a very early stage of the embryo's development. A process such as the closure of the neural tube happens on a specific day of the pregnancy — at a

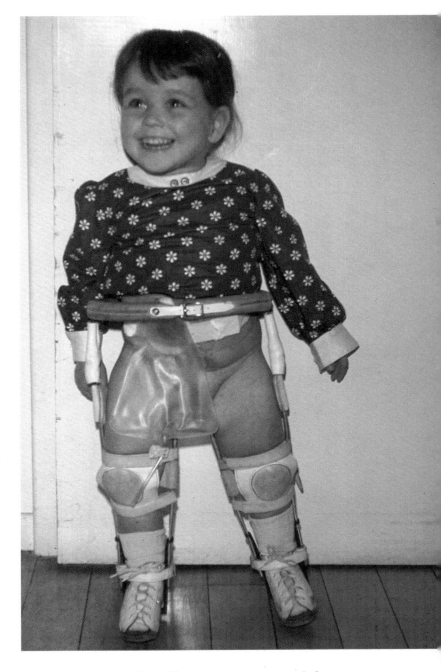

One of the most common congenital abnormalities is spina bifida. In the mildest cases the child suffers from weak limbs and can walk for short distances only with the aid of special supports.

113

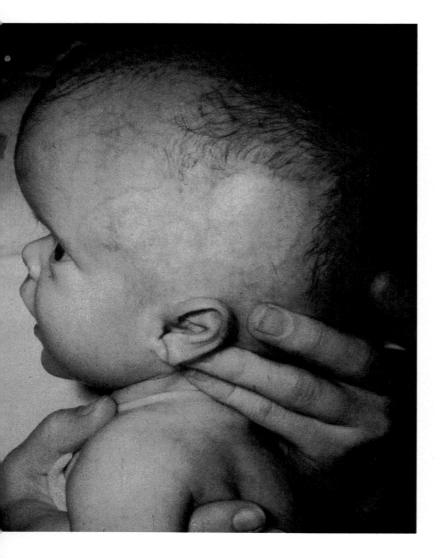

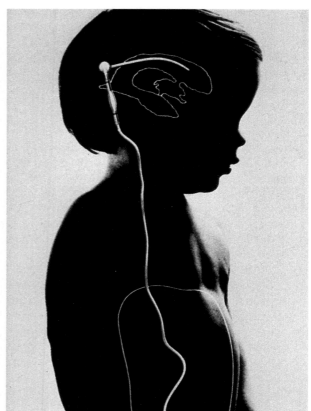

Hydrocephalus (left) *results from fluid accumulating in the cranial cavity. A shunt, or drainage system, can be installed* (below), *which channels the fluid into the abdomen where it is reabsorbed.*

stage when some women do not even know they are pregnant.

The claim has been made that these defects occur as a result of vitamin deficiency before conception and that, if all women of childbearing age regularly took folic acid, the incidence of spina bifida would be significantly reduced.

A researcher has examined regional diets and compared them with the incidence of spina bifida. Among a population that had a staple diet of potatoes, the rate of spina bifida was higher. The rate increased in babies conceived at the end of winter, and suspicion fell on green or blackened potatoes which had been stored for too long.

It is now possible to test a sample of blood during early pregnancy in order to detect signs of spina bifida in the embryo. If such signs are present, the woman has the choice of an abortion. This may be a satisfactory alternative for some women, but preconceptual prevention is undoubtedly a better

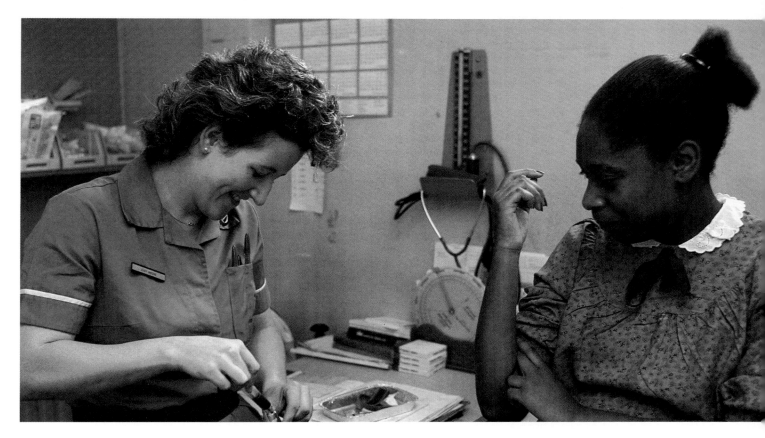

alternative, not necessarily from a moral viewpoint — although that is significant to many people — but particularly in view of the fact that abortion can have both physical and mental effects, some of which may be longlasting, on the woman involved. In any account, however, the choice between knowingly giving birth to a crippled baby or having an abortion may be agonizing. Providing a means to avoid such painful decisions at the preconceptual stage, therefore, is desirable.

The brain and spinal cord, in all their complexity, develop from just two cells. Within a forty-week period of intrauterine life they then go on to form networks of interconnecting fibers, and make almost endless connections with receptors and muscles throughout the body. Incredibly, the great majority of babies are born perfect in every detail, and continue to grow and develop into adults capable of great achievements in fields as diverse as sport, science, literature and philosophy.

Blood that is taken from a pregnant mother can be analyzed to discover indications of defects in the embryo, such as spina bifida or hydrocephaly. At an early stage she can then be given the option of an abortion.

115

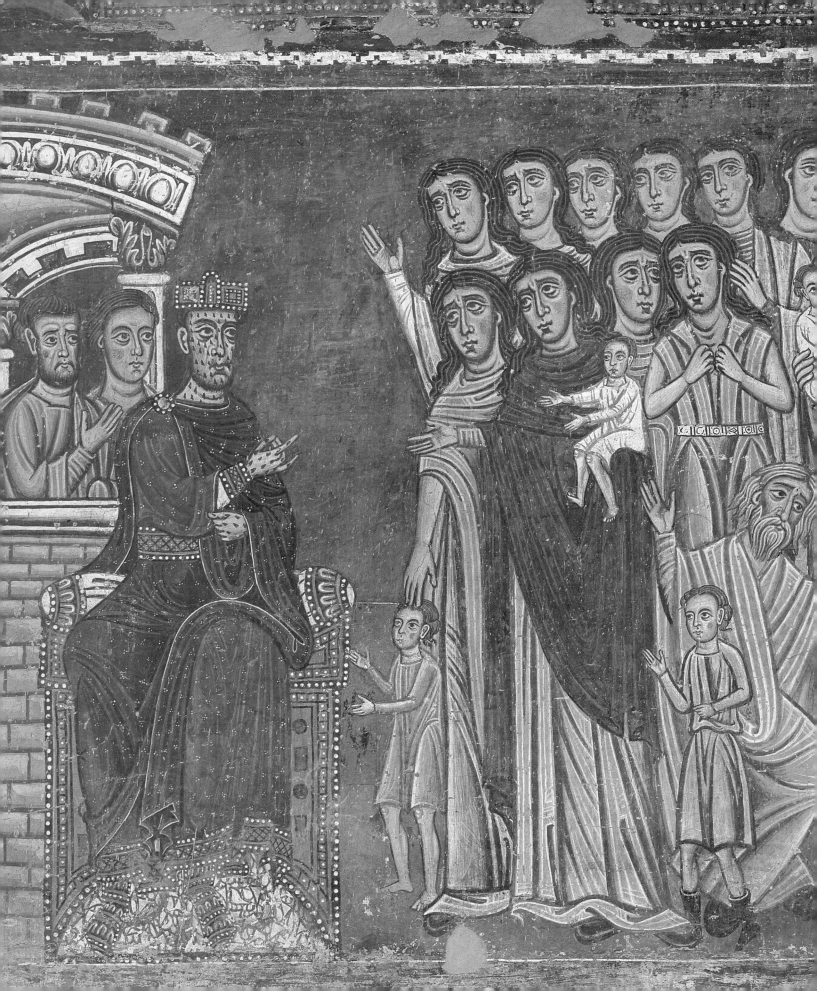

Chapter 7

Short Circuits in the System

Neurology is the study of the nervous system and the disorders that affect it. Physicians who specialize in treating such disorders are known as neurologists. Until the introduction of antibiotics, much of a neurologist's work was related to the once much more common disease of syphilis, in the later stages of which neurological complications occur. The first formal treatise on diseases of the nervous system was written by the German neurologist Moritz Romberg in 1846. At the same time there were also two great French neurologists: Guillaume Duchenne (1806–1875), who identified poliomyelitis as a disease that affected the spinal cord, and Jean-Martin Charcot (1825–1893), who accurately described the later stages of syphilis.

Until recently, neurology and psychiatry often were practised as the same speciality, and in some countries they still are. This is not surprising because the two branches of medicine overlap, especially in diseases causing degeneration of the brain. It has resulted in some confusion of terminology; the terms "nervy" or "nervous" are not infrequently used to describe emotional disorders rather than diseases of nerves.

Many people believe, erroneously, that diseases of the nervous system are incurable and always crippling. Although a few are, medical science has made great advances over the last 50 years in treating nervous diseases. Some diseases — such as polio — have been almost eliminated from the developed countries of the world, and effective treatments now exist for disorders such as syphilis and leprosy. Research is also progressing into diseases that are currently incurable, such as multiple sclerosis, and it is quite possible that effective treatments will become available in the near future.

This chapter considers the diseases that affect the nervous system. The object is to see how an understanding of anatomy and physiology can lead

A thirteenth-century fresco depicts Emperor Constantine I stricken with leprosy, although it is unlikely that he suffered from this disease but rather from a minor skin ailment. Leprosy, which affects the peripheral nervous system, was said to have been cured miraculously in Constantine's case. Today it is treated successfully with drugs.

117

Polio can now be monitored using computer graphics (below), which depict the contours of bones deformed as a consequence of muscle paralysis brought on by the disease. Vaccines against polio are well developed and can be given by mouth (oral vaccine); mixed in a sugary liquid or applied to a lump of sugar they are palatable and can easily be fed to babies. Vaccination has virtually eliminated polio in most developed countries.

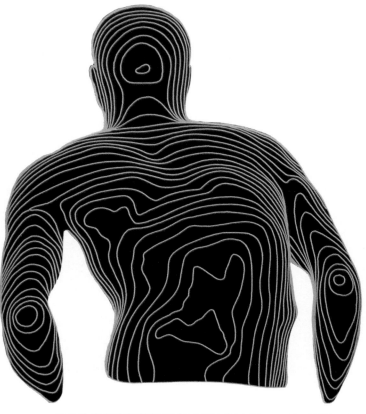

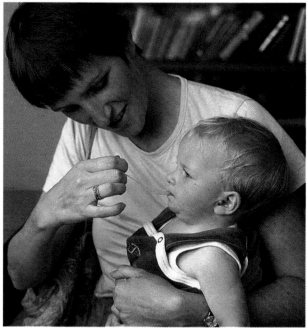

to effective treatments or can point the way to further research that may help conquer this group of disorders.

Viral Diseases

One of the great triumphs of modern medicine was the invention of an effective vaccine against polio. Poliomyelitis is caused by a group of closely related viruses which attack motor neurons in the anterior horns of the spinal cord and in the brainstem. The virus usually enters the body through the nasal passages or the gastrointestinal tract. It then travels in the bloodstream to the nervous system, and may invade peripheral nerves and travel up to the anterior horn cells.

Infected cells are destroyed. If the disease affects the motor neurons supplying muscles involved in breathing or swallowing, the patient's life is endangered. Sometimes the affected neurons recover and improvement may continue gradually over many months. Not all cases of polio progress to the paralytic stage, and the disease may stop at any of the earlier stages. However, many patients are left with residual disability.

Immunization against polio was introduced by the American microbiologist Jonas Salk in 1953. His vaccination involved repeated injection of a suspension containing inactivated (dead) virus of the three polio strains called Lansing, Brunhilde and Leon. Although the Salk vaccine made a major contribution to the control of polio, it has been largely replaced by the Sabin vaccine, developed by Albert Sabin and first used in the United States in 1960. This consists of live viruses that have been weakened, and so do not produce any illness but stimulate the body to produce antibodies to polio viruses. The Sabin vaccine is active when taken by mouth, is cheaper to prepare and is more effective than the Salk vaccine.

Another viral disease that affects the human nervous system is rabies. All mammals can be affected by this disease, although vampire bats are unique in that they carry the virus and yet do not suffer from the disease. In humans, rabies is caused by a bite from an infected animal, usually a dog or other small carnivore. In the United States a number of victims are hunters who wound a small animal and are then bitten while trying to capture

Poliomyelitis is a viral disease which enters the body through the mouth and nose and passes to the lungs (1). From there it gets into the bloodstream (2) and disperses, eventually affecting the peripheral nervous system (3). Paralysis (4) occurs most frequently in the legs and more rarely in the arms. The least common form of the disease affects the brain. This type, bulbar spinal polio, is characterized by constricted capillaries in the spinal cord which leads to congestion in the anterior horn cells. The mitochondria of these cells deteriorate and the nuclei shrink and eventually the cells degenerate.

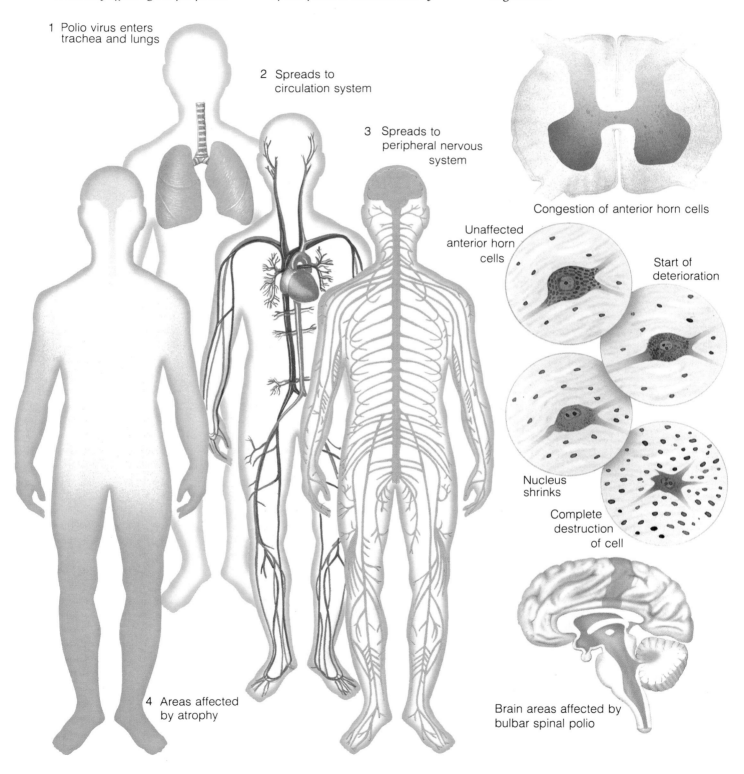

1 Polio virus enters trachea and lungs

2 Spreads to circulation system

3 Spreads to peripheral nervous system

4 Areas affected by atrophy

Congestion of anterior horn cells

Unaffected anterior horn cells

Start of deterioration

Nucleus shrinks

Complete destruction of cell

Brain areas affected by bulbar spinal polio

Rabies is usually contracted from the bite of a rabid mammal, such as a dog. The disease affects the central and peripheral nervous systems and is fatal if not treated in its early stages, before symptoms develop.

Shingles is caused by the virus Herpes zoster, which attacks the skin and its nerve endings. It is extremely painful and is characterized by small blisters which appear in the region of skin supplied by the affected nerve.

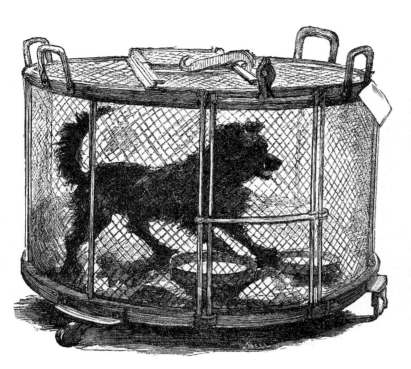

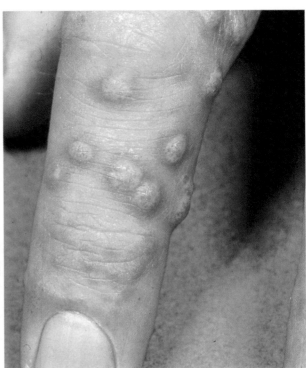

it. The rabies virus enters the nervous system along the peripheral nerves and attacks the nerve cells of the spinal cord and brain. In humans, the disease incubates for 28 to 60 days, and appropriate vaccination during this period prevents it. Hydrophobia (fear of water) is a common symptom; any attempt to drink brings on spasms which involve the muscles of respiration and those of the trunk and limbs.

A common viral infection of the nervous system is shingles, caused by infection of a posterior root ganglion by *Herpes zoster*. This virus is identical to the one which causes chickenpox. Following infection with chickenpox, the virus remains latent in the nervous system, often for years. If it is reactivated, the symptoms are marked by a dull pain along the distribution of the affected nerve roots — generally represented on the skin surface by the affected dermatome, a horizontal strip of skin around one side of the body. This is followed in a few days by a rash with vesicles similar to the lesions of chickenpox. The initial period of the rash may be followed by severe and lasting pain.

Bacterial Diseases

Another neurological disease that has been effectively controlled by immunization is tetanus (or lockjaw). Tetanus follows infection with the bacterium *Clostridium tetani*, found in the soil. The bacterium enters the body through wounds such as cuts or punctures—the initial injury may be quite minor. The organism multiplies only under anaerobic conditions (without oxygen). Anaerobic conditions are likely to occur in deep penetrating wounds, such as those caused by stepping on a nail. The bacteria multiply and produce a toxin (a powerful poison) which attacks motor nerves and anterior horn cells. If the anterior horn cells are affected, muscle rigidity and spasm follow. The incubation period is from two days to several weeks and a common early symptom is spasm of the jaw muscles, which causes difficulty in opening the mouth and gives the disease its common name, lockjaw.

At the end of the last century, the German bacteriologist Emil von Behring produced a toxoid for active immunization against tetanus. Toxoids

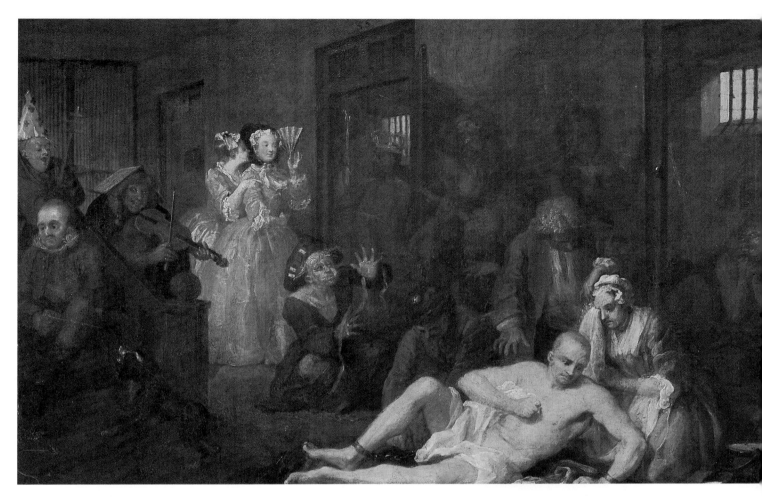

are produced by purifying the toxin and inactivating it with heat and formalin. This renders the toxin harmless, but the toxoid so produced stimulates antibody production against the toxin. Active immunization against tetanus is carried out on most children in the United States, and "booster" injections are often given as added protection for individuals who have suffered a potentially dangerous wound.

The success of medical science against syphilis has been attained through effective treatment rather than the development of a vaccine. Syphilis is caused by infection with a bacterium, a spirochaete called *Treponema pallidum*. Neurological manifestations of the disease do not occur until many years after the original infection. Penicillins are now used to treat this disease, generally arresting its development in the primary or secondary stages before neurological symptoms have developed. Even if given later in the course of the disease, penicillins also usually arrest the development of further neurological symptoms.

Leprosy, the most common infectious neuro-

Hogarth's moralizing series of paintings which recounts the physical and moral decline of a rake ends with the debauched man, demented by syphilis and housed in an asylum, overlooked by sightseers. Dementia paralytica, a form of neurosyphilis, affects the brain and spinal cord, inflaming and shriveling their cells. Syphilis can now be treated successfully with antibiotics such as penicillin.

Multiple sclerosis is, at present, an incurable disease which destroys the myelin sheath of nerve fibers in the brain, hindering the conduction of impulses. It weakens the limbs forcing victims to be chairbound.

Multiple Sclerosis

The cause of multiple sclerosis remains unknown, although various theories exist. The disease often affects more than one member of a family, indicating that there may be a genetic disposition toward it. Theories include that the disease is caused by excessive animal fat in the diet, by heavy-metal poisoning or by venous thrombosis. It is also possible that the nervous system is hypersensitive to one or more common viruses, such as the measles virus. Measles is implicated because more than 90 per cent of multiple sclerosis patients have high concentrations of antibodies to the measles virus in their cerebrospinal fluid.

Another possibility is that multiple sclerosis is caused by a "slow virus" which is acquired in childhood and takes many years to produce symptoms. Yet another possibility is that multiple sclerosis is an autoimmune disease; that is, a malfunction of the immune system so that the body reacts against part of itself. Immune cells (lymphocytes and plasma cells) have been found in the patches of demyelination around affected nerves. Although the cause of this disease eludes medical knowledge, it is possible that research in one of the areas mentioned will soon prove fruitful.

Multiple sclerosis commonly occurs in episodes or waves; first one part of the nervous system and then another is affected and then recovers. It is the characteristic relapsing and remitting nature of the disease that allows the diagnosis to be made. A common first symptom is visual disturbance, with blurring and dimming of vision accompanied by pain in the eye. Often there is partial or complete recovery within a few days or weeks. Other symptoms may be weakness or loss of control in one or more limbs. Alternatively, there may be loss of sensation, with tingling or numbness in an affected area. When behavior or consciousness is affected — usually a late sign — speech may become slurred and the patient may become euphoric. The individual appears exceptionally cheerful and unconcerned about an obvious disability.

It is not possible to predict the course of multiple sclerosis. An attack may clear up completely, and the individual may be free from symptoms for many months or years (remission), or for ever. Alternatively, there may be repeated episodes

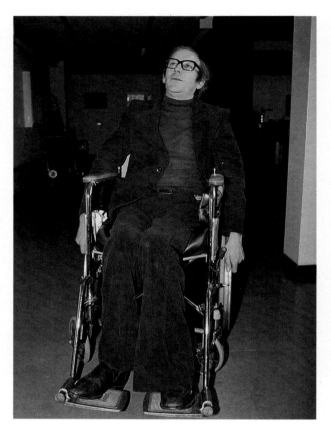

logical disease, is often curable, contrary to popular belief. The disease affects some 15 million people, mainly in tropical and subtropical countries. Leprosy is caused by a bacterium, *Mycobacterium leprae*, which affects individual peripheral nerves and causes them to become thickened. Sensation is lost in parts of the body supplied by these nerves, and skin and bone become damaged. This often leads to marked deformities of the feet, hands and face. Leprosy is far less infectious than was once thought, and treatment with dapsone — introduced in 1944 — is effective, but it must be continued for many years.

The term demyelinating disease comprises a group of neurological disorders of which multiple sclerosis is the commonest example. Demyelination describes the loss of the myelin sheath from a nerve. Without myelin the fiber cannot conduct impulses properly, so that the function served by the nerve is disturbed.

The vagus is the tenth cranial nerve and is the only cranial nerve to extend through the body as far as the visceral parts. Many diseases with a psychosomatic element often affect the organs supplied by this nerve,

suggesting a possible link between vagal stimulation and psychological factors. Symptoms of disordered vagal function include poor digestion, which results from slowed movement of food through the gut

due to reduced peristalsis as well as to reduced secretion of digestive enzymes, loss of reflex control in the circulatory system, which upsets the heart rate and blood pressure, and problems with swallowing or speech.

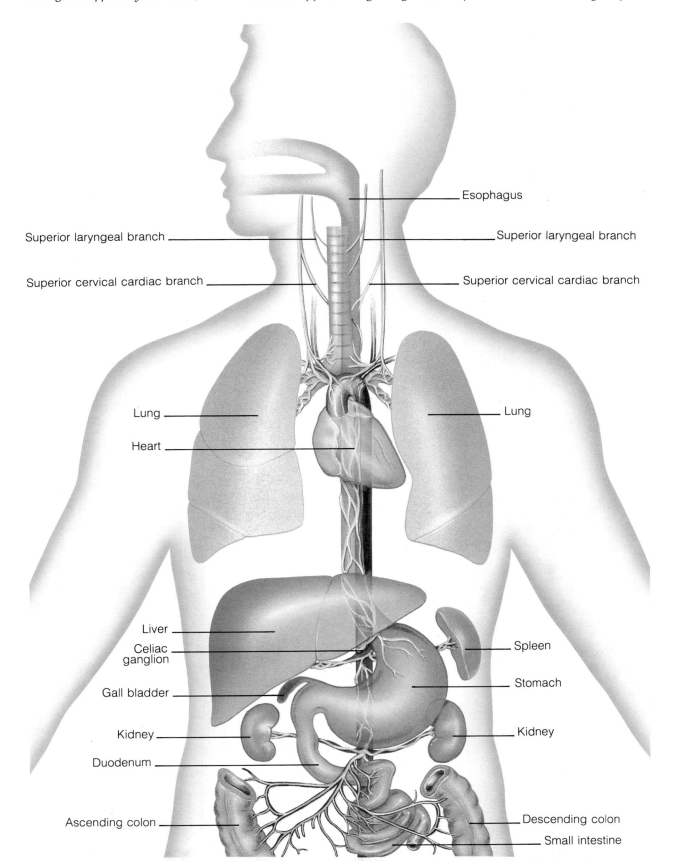

Esophagus

Superior laryngeal branch

Superior laryngeal branch

Superior cervical cardiac branch

Superior cervical cardiac branch

Lung

Lung

Heart

Liver

Spleen

Celiac ganglion

Stomach

Gall bladder

Kidney

Kidney

Duodenum

Ascending colon

Descending colon

Small intestine

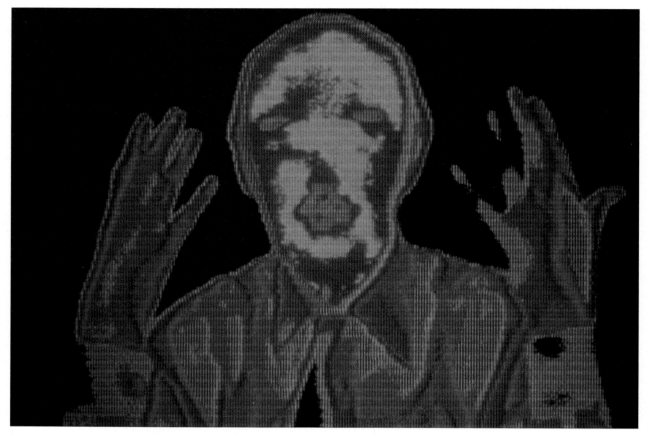

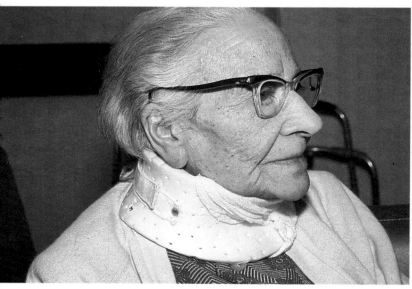

The degeneration of joint surfaces in the cervical column can lead to spinal cord compression and severe pain. Mild cases can be treated with a cervical collar, which keeps the neck still and reduces the pain.

(relapses), affecting different parts of the nervous system. If there are many closely linked relapses, the outlook is less favourable than if attacks are widely spaced in time. No cure for the disease has been found.

Because of the relapsing and remitting nature of multiple sclerosis, it is difficult even to assess the results of treatment. Steroid drugs have sometimes been successful in treating acute relapses. Injections of either cortisone or adrenocorticotropic hormone (ACTH), are given to stimulate the body to produce its own steroids. The benefits are transient. Various dietary treatments — including gluten-free diets and diets rich in sunflower seeds — have been tried without benefit. Treatment with oxygen in a compression chamber — hyperbaric oxygen treatment — has produced transient improvement in some patients. Immunosuppressive treatments with anti-cancer drugs have been reported to produce more longlasting benefits, but at the cost of an increased risk of infection and of malignancy in later life.

Cord Compression Disorders

One group of neurological disorders amenable to treatment are those caused by compression of the spinal cord, nerve roots or peripheral nerves. The spinal cord may be compressed by a prolapsed intervertebral disk (slipped disk), or by a crush fracture of a vertebral bone. Disk displacement is a common cause of the lower back pain lumbago or the pain in the upper leg known as sciatica. Metastatic cancer affecting the vertebrae can compress the spinal cord; cancers of the breast, prostate and lung may cause this problem.

Tuberculosis of the spine (Pott's disease) was once a common cause of spinal cord compression but is now rare outside of developing countries. Primary tumors of the spinal cord itself may also give rise to symptoms of cord compression. The effects of compression arise because of direct pressure damage to the spinal cord or the nerve or because of pressure on the arteries and veins which supply them. If the arteries or veins are obstructed, the nervous tissue is deprived of its oxygen and glucose supply, and dies. Osteoarthritis is a condition that commonly affects the vertebral column, particularly in the neck, and may cause symptoms of spinal cord, spinal nerve root, and peripheral nerve compression. In rare cases, the arthritic overgrowth of bone can compress the whole of the spinal cord.

Cervical arthritis with compression of the spinal cord or spinal nerves, a common problem in the elderly, is termed cervical spondylosis. If there are signs of acute cervical root compression, characterized by pain and tingling in the arms and hands, but no signs of acute cord compression — indicated by spasticity and weakness of the legs, with numbness and tingling in the feet — then cervical spondylosis is usually treated with immobilization using a cervical collar, and rest. Signs of acute cord compression require surgical intervention. Before surgery, the site and extent of cord compression must be identified. This is done by means of a special X-ray examination called a myelogram, in which a radiopaque fluid that shows up on X-ray film is injected into the cerebrospinal fluid. This enables a protruding disk or bone spur to be seen easily, and shows the surgeon exactly where to operate. A myelogram is necessary to localize the position and extent of spinal cord tumors so that they can be treated by surgical removal if benign or by radiation treatment if malignant.

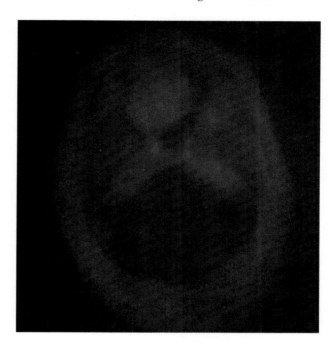

Recently, other techniques have become available to help locate cord lesions. One is CAT scanning (computed axial tomography), which can locate damage very precisely. An even newer procedure, magnetic resonance imaging (MRI) also holds great promise, and may replace myelography as an investigative technique.

Lesions and Traumas

Impaired conduction in peripheral nerves may be reversible or irreversible. Neuropraxis describes a condition in which nerve conduction is blocked in a reversible manner, with subsequent full recovery. By contrast, neurotomesis means that the continuity of the fibers has been interrupted so that they subsequently degenerate. A total lesion of a mixed sensory and motor nerve results in paralysis of the muscles supplied by the nerve, which then waste away; at the same time there is an absence of sensation over the area (dermatome) supplied by the nerve. The area of loss of sensation is often less than might be expected because the dermatomes supplied by sensory nerves overlap in their distribution.

Until recently, severing of nerves was the only treatment for some forms of neuralgia. This was

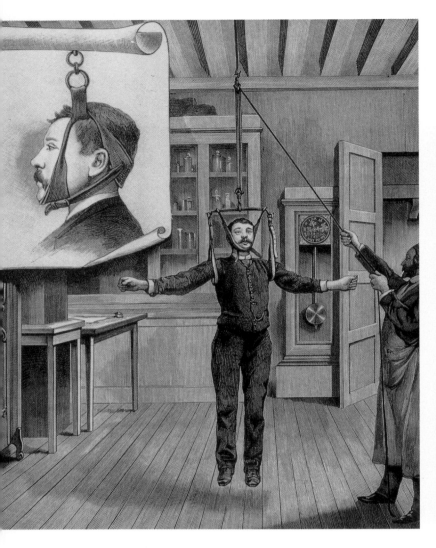

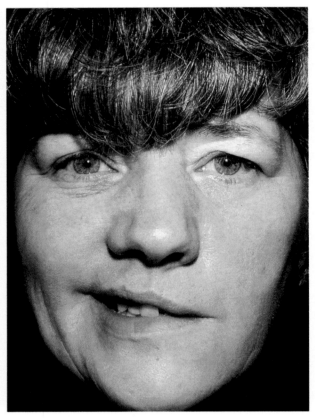

The lack of muscular coordination symptomatic of ataxia was treated in the 1890s by Dr Stein's harness (left). Similarly a splint is used to support drooping facial muscles paralyzed by Bell's palsy (below).

true particularly of trigeminal neuralgia (tic douleureux) in one side of the face — surgery tended to leave numb areas. Today, treatment of tic with drugs, such as the anticonvulsant carpamazepine, often is successful. After any serious surface wound, numbness of the area around the wound occurs and then gradually disappears.

Groups of nerves, or plexuses, may also be affected by compression or trauma. The brachial plexus, which contains all the nerves from the spinal cord to the arm, is often injured or compressed when a person falls onto one shoulder. A fracture of the head of the humerus, the upper arm bone, may also damage the brachial plexus. Severe injuries involving downward movement of the shoulder may even tear the spinal nerves out of the spinal cord.

A common form of peripheral nerve entrapment, to which middle-aged women are particularly prone, occurs in the wrist and is called carpal tunnel syndrome. Injury to the median nerve in the carpal tunnel may result from excessive movement of the wrist, as in piano playing or knitting. The tendon sheaths of the flexor muscles of the hand swell and the median nerve is compressed underneath the carpal ligament in the wrist. Typical symptoms of median nerve compression are pain, burning, or a tingling sensation in the first and second fingers. The symptoms are usually worse at night. This common syndrome is easily cured by surgical division of the ligament.

Neurofibromatosis and Neuromuscular Disorders

Neurofibromatosis, or Von Recklinghausen's disease, is inherited as an autosomal dominant trait, that is, through the presence of a single abnormal gene. The disease is associated with patchy increased pigmentation of the skin, described as ''café au lait'' spots. Affected persons suffer from multiple tumors which grow from the

126

One of the most important nerves in the wrist is the median nerve, which connects with the muscles of the thumb and innervates it and the first two fingers (below). This nerve passes through the carpal tunnel, which contains soft tissue and fat. Carpal tunnel syndrome results when the tissue becomes swollen and compresses the median nerve, causing intense pain, a burning sensation and tingling in the hand, particularly at night. If it is not treated, the muscles in the hand may waste. The condition is common in middle-aged women who use their hands often in such activities as spinning or weaving (bottom).

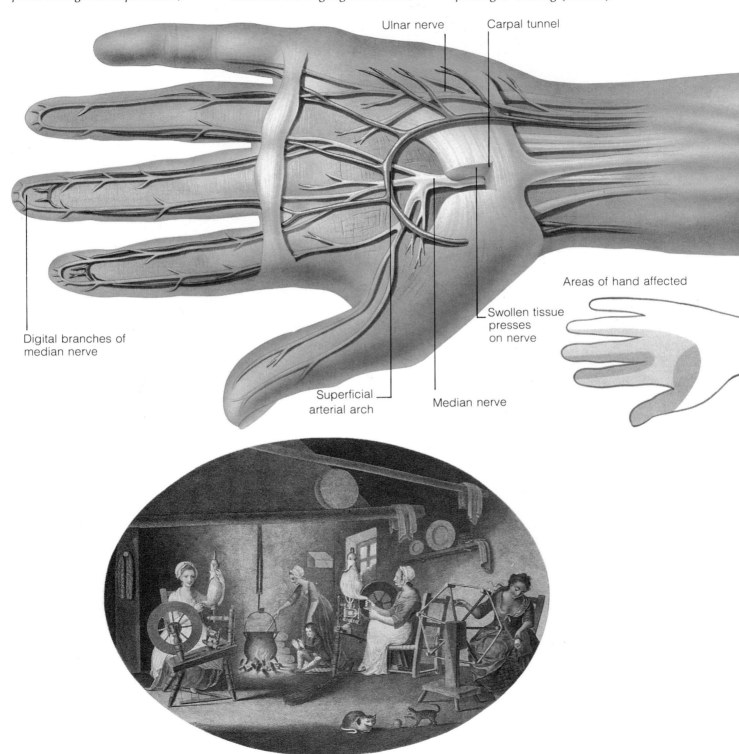

Ulnar nerve

Carpal tunnel

Areas of hand affected

Swollen tissue presses on nerve

Digital branches of median nerve

Superficial arterial arch

Median nerve

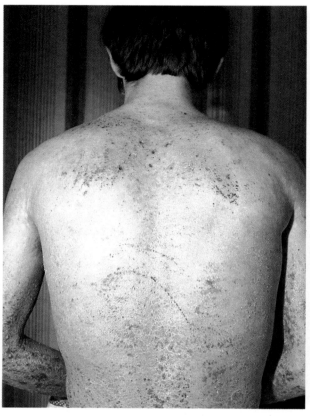

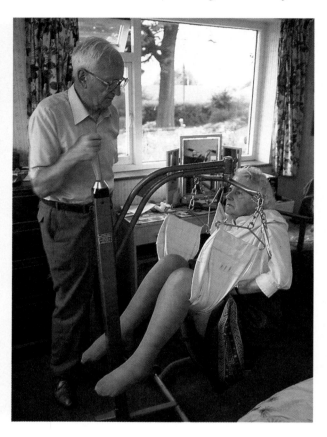

sheaths of the nerves. These tumors are generally benign, although malignant change may occur. Lesions under the skin cause many swellings; these neurofibromas may also cause nerve compression. Surgery is sometimes used to remove the lumps, and many sufferers of the disease live on to an old age. Sometimes the skin over the lumps can assume the characteristics of elephant skin, and it is likely that the Elephant Man — whose story has been shown on film and the stage — suffered from this.

There is a group of neuromuscular diseases called myotonias, in which muscles do not relax after a contraction. After taking hold of an object, it may take several seconds for the fingers to relax and let it go. The cause of myotonia is unclear. It is thought that a disturbance in chloride conduction in the muscle fiber membrane might be responsible.

There are two main types of myotonia, both inherited as dominant traits. Myotonia congenita is present from birth, and affected infants may experience difficulty in crying and feeding. Most muscle groups may be affected and may grow abnormally large (hypertrophy). Persons affected have a normal lifespan. The other type, dystrophia myotonica, usually comes on later, in late adolescence or adulthood, and generally affects mainly the hands and tongue. Patients develop frontal baldness, and some of the muscles of the head, such as the temporals, and of the neck, such as the sternomastoids, become thin and wasted. The disease progresses slowly until the patient is wheelchair-bound in later life. Various medications, including steroid therapy, are available to relieve myotonia.

Neuropathies and Autoimmune Disorders

One of the most benign of the familial neurological disorders, peroneal muscular atrophy, or Charcot-Marie-Tooth disease, usually develops in early adult life. The patient develops muscular atrophy

Jean-Martin Charcot

The Mind-Body Link

Drama and eloquence were two major features in the teaching of Jean-Martin Charcot, the French pioneer in medical treatments based on the new science of neurology. So celebrated were his lectures, which were delivered with rhetorical passion on a small stage, that students came from all over the world to see and hear him.

Born in Paris in 1825, Charcot became Professor of Pathological Anatomy at Paris University at the age of only 35, after studying there himself. Two years later, there began an association between Charcot and the Salpêtrière Hospital in Paris that was to be remarkable and formative for both the hospital and Charcot.

Charcot's strength and genius were founded on a novel approach to his subject that was both holistic (relating the nervous system to every part of the body and its disorders) and zonal (apprehending that there were nevertheless different parts of the nervous system that had different functions). His synthesis of these previously incompatible ideas also included the use of pathological criteria in diagnoses of nervous disorders.

In 1882 Charcot opened his

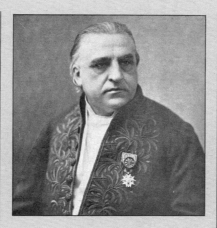

own clinic at the Salpêtrière Hospital, becoming Professor of Neurology there while remaining Professor of Medicine at the University. His great interest at this time was the link between the body and the mind, a study which led to his major achievement, which was to provide a scientific understanding of hysteria and hypnotic states. These conditions were distinguished from organic malfunctions or diseases, and Charcot showed that they could be diagnosed by specific signs and symptoms.

Charcot was the first to describe in detail nervous conditions such as tabes dorsalis (a type of late or tertiary syphilis), motor neuron disease (ALS), and multiple sclerosis. He also initiated the investigation of the effects of the loss of pain perception

from joints in patients with tabes dorsalis. Painless trauma led, in these patients, to the degeneration of ligaments and joint surfaces (now known as Charcot's disease of joints).

Charcot was a great believer in the efficacy of hypnosis in treatment, and made good use of it with his patients. From being the province of sideshows and drawing-room parties, hypnosis rapidly came to have scientific credibility and status. The best known of Charcot's students to be influenced by this innovation was Sigmund Freud.

Charcot also studied cerebral localization, and contributed to contemporary scientific attempts to determine which physical areas of the brain controlled specific activities or sensitivities. In carrying out this work he discovered and described a certain type of aneurysm (swelling of the wall of an artery) significant as a cause of cerebral hemorrhage in patients with untreated hypertension.

A man of great visual sensibilities, Charcot was also concerned to promote the depiction of medical studies in art. Author, innovator and, above all, teacher, he died in 1893. In retrospect, he is regarded as the founder of modern neurology.

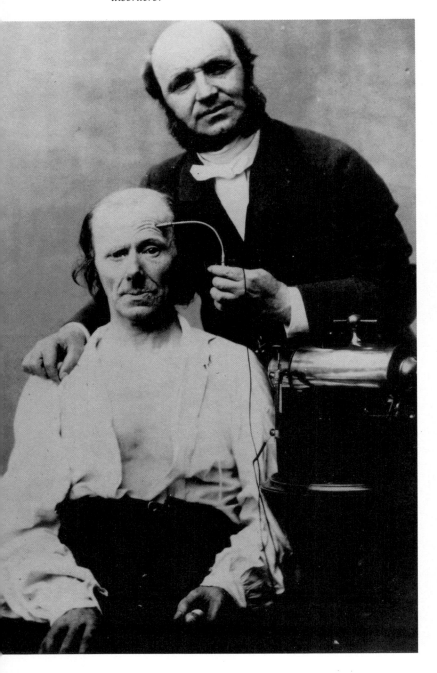

(wasting) and weakness. The muscles of the leg are affected, although patients remain active into later life. The disease is caused by changes in the motor neurons or peripheral nerves. Therefore, in spite of its name, the disease is a neuropathy, a disease of nerves, rather than a myopathy, a disease of muscles. The pattern of muscle wasting, which is localized and stops mid-thigh, gives the legs a characteristic appearance known as champagne-bottle thighs. The muscles of the forearm and hand are affected later in the course of the disease.

Another large group of neurological diseases affects the motor neurons and muscles. Some are amenable to effective treatment, but others are incurable and progressive; an accurate early diagnosis is thus essential. Motor neuron disease usually begins after the age of forty. The primary disorder is a degeneration of motor neurons in the spinal cord leading to progressive weakness, often beginning in the hands or shoulders. As the condition spreads, there is muscle wasting throughout the body. The trunk no longer gives support, and the gradual weakness of the throat and tongue muscles impairs swallowing and speech. Death occurs in a few years, usually from respiratory insufficiency and pneumonia. The cause of motor neuron disease is uncertain and no treatment is known.

Myasthenia gravis is a disease which affects the neuromuscular junction where the motor neuron makes contact with and delivers signals to muscle fibers. The disease is a type of autoimmune process in which the immune system makes antibodies which react with the receptors for the neurotransmitter acetylcholine on the muscle cell membrane. As a result, the number of receptors is greatly reduced and the muscle can only "receive" a limited number of nerve impulses before its supply of receptors is used up. In some patients the autoimmune reaction is due to a tumor of the thymus gland, and can be successfully treated by surgical removal of the thymus.

The disease usually starts between the ages of fifteen and fifty, and is more common in women than in men. The effect is the same as that produced by curare, the arrow poison of South American Indians. The muscles of respiration may eventually become involved, and death may result from

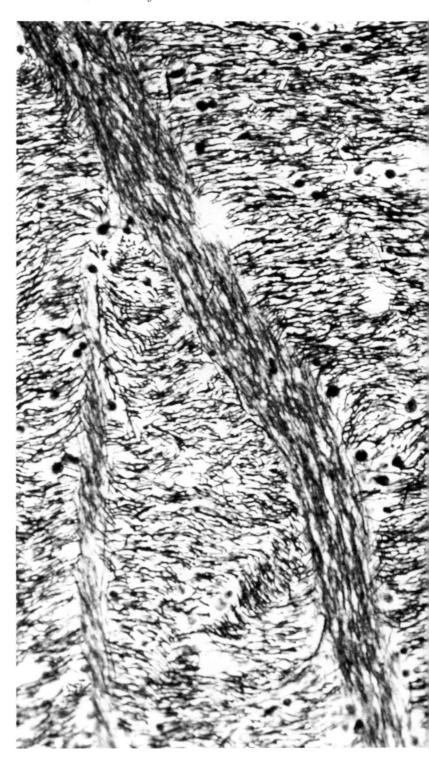

respiratory failure. There is, however, an effective treatment for the muscle weakness. The neurotransmitter acetylcholine is normally broken down and rendered ineffective after its release by an enzyme called cholinesterase. Patients suffering from myasthenia gravis are given the drug neostigmine, which inhibits the effect of cholinesterase and increases the amount of acetylcholine available to the muscle receptors. Corticosteroids may inhibit the autoimmune process, and plasmapheresis—by washing the patient's serum clean of antibodies—also is helpful.

It is important to help the myasthenic patient to manage life in a way that avoids stress and reduces fatigue. The outcome for any one case of myasthenia gravis is impossible to predict accurately.

There are forms of peripheral neuropathy in which several peripheral nerves are involved simultaneously. A form of ascending paralysis is called the Guillain-Barre syndrome. Paralysis usually follows an infective illness but may arise on its own. There is weakness, generally starting in the limb muscles, which spreads (within hours or days) to involve the muscles of the trunk and respiration. Supportive therapy is necessary and may, if the muscles of respiration are involved, require artificial ventilation in an intensive care unit. This syndrome is interesting because the disease usually resolves spontaneously. The symptoms gradually decline over a period of months, and the patient recovers completely.

Guillain-Barre syndrome is a disease of the autoimmune type, in which an inflammatory response occurs within the nerves. Immune cells damage the myelin around the nerve but do not destroy the nerve itself, so that eventually it recovers. Recently, a vaccine against swine influenza caused an epidemic of Guillain-Barre syndrome among the recipients in the United States.

There are various other types of peripheral neuropathy, which are generally of mixed motor and sensory type. This means that as well as the motor system's becoming involved and producing weakness or paralysis, there is loss of sensation in the affected areas. Causes include infections such as leprosy, infectious mononucleosis (glandular fever), typhoid and dysentery. Neuropathies may occur in association with various forms of malig-

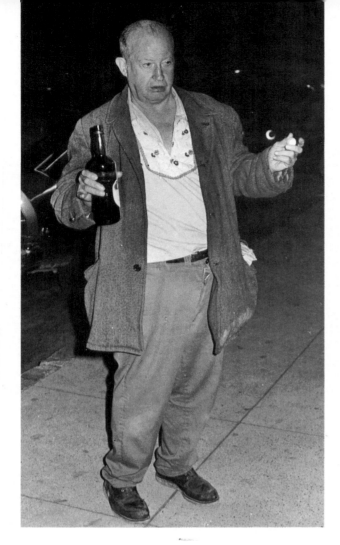

nant disease for reasons that are not understood. Diseases involving abnormal immune responses, such as systemic lupus erythematosus or polyarteritis nodosa, often are associated with neuropathies.

Metabolic Disorders

A final group of nervous system diseases are those related to metabolic disorders. Alterations in metabolic activity, whether due to vitamin deficiency or hormonal disorders, may lead to nervous system changes. Dietary deficiency of thiamine (vitamin B_1) leads to beriberi. The commonest cause of thiamine deficiency, neuropathy occurs in chronic alcoholics, who often do not eat normal meals and suffer from deficiencies of many vitamins. The principal result of thiamine deficiency is polyneuropathy. In addition to muscular weakness and sensory loss, occurring with all neuropathies, affected subjects often complain of intense burning and tingling in the hands and feet. (It is estimated that the United States could save $100–$300 million a year in medical costs if thiamine was added to alcoholic drinks to prevent alcohol-related thiamine deficiency disorders.) A similar syndrome occurred in prisoner-of-war camps during World War II — burning feet syndrome. Prisoners complained of agonizing burning of the feet, but this occurred without any signs of motor neuropathy. The syndrome responded to high doses of B vitamins.

Another vitamin deficiency that causes neurological symptoms is B_{12} deficiency. Dietary deficiency of B_{12} is rare, and occurs only in very strict vegetarians, called Vegans. The deficiency usually is revealed by pernicious anemia, in which a substance called intrinsic factor is absent from the gastric juices. Dietary intake of B_{12} may be adequate, but without intrinsic factor it cannot be absorbed. Because intrinsic factor is produced by the gastric mucosa, B_{12} deficiency can also occur after surgery in which a large part of the stomach is removed.

The neurological syndrome produced by B_{12} deficiency is called subacute combined degeneration of the spinal cord, because the posterior columns (sensory tract) and the corticospinal (motor) tracts of the spinal cord are affected, along with posterior nerve roots and peripheral nerves. There is a loss of myelin and degeneration of nerve axons. The initial symptoms are tingling and numbness. If the corticospinal tracts are affected, there is disturbed motor function, with stiffness and slowness of walking. Patients with pernicious anemia or who have had a gastrectomy (removal of the stomach) are treated with B_{12} injections to prevent subacute combined denudation of the spinal cord.

Diseases of the endocrine system, particularly diabetes mellitus, also may cause neuropathies. Diabetes is caused by a deficiency of insulin, a hormone secreted in the pancreas, which controls the blood sugar level. Treatment therefore includes diet control or, in severe cases, daily injections of insulin. Diabetic polyneuropathy occurs when the blood sugar level has been too high for a long time. The exact cause is unknown, and it does not respond to insulin treatment. Symptoms are mainly sensory, with burning in the hands and feet. There may be an associated difficulty in walking.

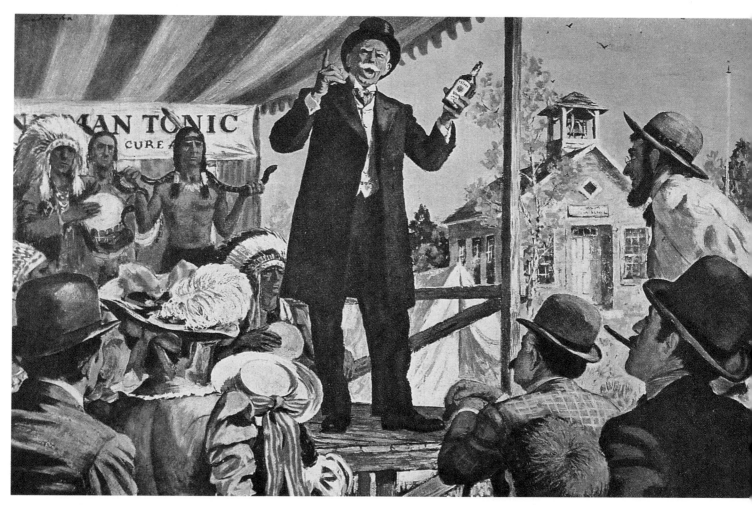

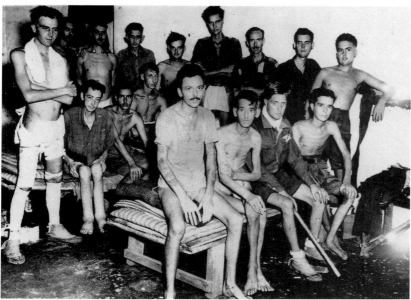

The Medicine Man (above) exploited the gullibility of his onlookers by boldly selling "nerve tonics," which were guaranteed to restore calm and rejuvenate. Many of the tonics contained cocaine, alcohol or opium, which induced a misleading and temporary euphoria and so seemed to reduce depression and anxiety. Such emotions are frequently caused by vitamin deficiencies, and were experienced by prisoners of war (left), exaggerating their already low morale. Their neurological deterioration manifested itself in reduced ability to feel touch, and in burning or tingling feelings in their hands and feet.

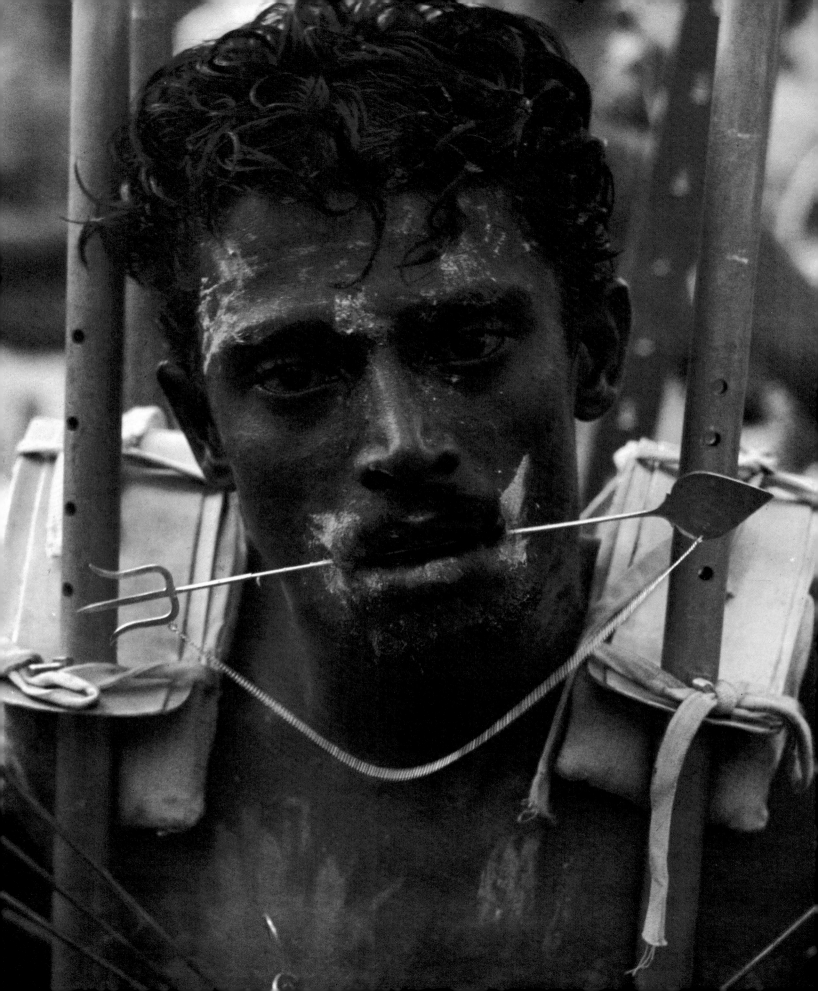

Chapter 8

Agony and Ecstasy

Pain is something that is never welcomed yet it is important in enabling the body to be protected from injury. The appreciation of a painful sensation and the response to it are complicated. Consider the sensation of heat. Sitting in a swimsuit in the sun on a warm day can be a pleasant and comfortable sensation. But if the day is very hot then the sensation can be somewhat uncomfortable.

Skin exposed for too long becomes painful and burned. In response to the stimulus of the sun the person can turn over in order to protect the hot part of the body from the sun or, at a certain level of discomfort, can move away into the shade. The nervous pathways involved in the integration of such a response are complex, and some of them are explored in this chapter.

Pain may act as a warning and be valuable to the person feeling the pain. Another example is the pain of angina pectoris, which occurs when the blood vessels to the heart are narrowed. During exercise, the heart uses more oxygen, and when the narrowed arteries cannot supply enough oxygen-carrying blood, chest pain or angina is felt. Pain warns the person to stop exercising and allow the heart a rest; otherwise a heart attack (myocardial infarction) may occur. The treatment of this pain is not to use analgesics (pain-relieving drugs) but to use other medications which encourage more blood to get to the heart.

Pain as a warning also occurs as the acute pain that is felt when a bone is broken. Such pain prevents the sufferer from moving the limb and doing further damage. Immobilization or splinting of an injured limb often reduces the pain.

Pain is not always beneficial, of course, and the pain that occurs with some types of cancer and following surgery are examples of this. Physicians now have many drugs to relieve pain, and by using them appropriately fulfil one of their most important functions to benefit humankind.

As part of a Hindu religious festival this Malaysian tribesman has allowed a steel spike to be driven through his cheeks. His trancelike expression betrays no indication of pain. Attitude of mind, therefore, would seem to be all important if pain is successfully to be ignored.

135

Treatment of pain also has important economic implications. Chronic pain caused by backache or arthritis is the most common cause of inability to work; the cost both in lost production and in medical care is enormous.

How Pain Is Felt

Perception of painful stimuli occurs via peripheral nerves which conduct the information to the brain via the spinal cord. Peripheral neurons called first-order neurons, at the site of the original stimulus, synapse in the dorsal horns of the spinal cord; the second-order neurons pick up the signal, take it over to the other side of the spinal cord, and pass it upward in the spinothalamic tracts to the thalamus of the brain. This fast-conducting pathway is for the perception of sharp or acute pain.

An alternative pathway exists in which the second-order neurons are represented by a series of interconnected neurons; this slow-ascending pathway allows perception of duller, more persistent pain. These pain pathways travel up the spinal cord to connect with the brainstem (the medulla and the midbrain), the thalamus, and then the cerebral cortex. There is a third pathway formed by large myelinated fibers which travel in the dorsal columns of the spinal cord. The function of this pathway is unclear, but may be related to fine discrimination or vibration sense.

Two types of neuron are concerned with pain perception entering the spinal cord: the A delta group and unmyelinated C fibers. Each type has a different pathway for transmission to the central nervous system. The A delta fibers are those concerned with the perception of sharp pain; the unmyelinated C fibers are much more numerous than the A delta fibers, and are responsible for transmitting dull, persistent pain.

The autonomic or involuntary nervous system is also involved in the perception of pain. It functions without conscious control and affects the heart, the gut, and the blood vessels. For pain, its afferent pathway to the brain is similar to that of the multiple ascending system (MAS) of the unmyelinated C fibers, but in fact there are few sensory nerves to the internal organs, with the result that most internal pain is poorly localized, dull and persistent in nature. This is not true of all visceral pain. Pain from the heart and kidney is characteristic, and allows the clinician to localize the affected area accurately.

The mechanism by which various unpleasant stimulations give rise to pain has been studied by scientists for centuries. Stimulation — such as touch or pressure, heat or cold — always gives rise to the same sensation. Only when the stimulation is above a certain level does the uniform sensation of pain occur. In the second half of the nineteenth century von Frey proposed a theory that each separate sensory modality had its own particular receptor. Various research workers of the time supported this theory by supposedly identifying the receptors in the skin and attaching their own names to them. This led to the discovery of Meissner's corpuscles for touch sensation, the cold bulb of Drause, and the heat organ of Ruffini. Pain was thought to arise from stimulation of a network of small nerve fibers.

A second theory of the mechanism for perceiving pain was proposed which related pain only to the intensity of stimulation — pain could arise from any form of external stimulation as long as it was powerful enough. In fact, elements in both theories are correct. The sensory theory, involving specific receptors, was put in doubt by the failure of scientists to prove the existence of a network of small nerve fibers and receptors with the high degree of specificity required by the theory. (However it has already been seen that there is some degree of specificity in pain perception, the A delta fibers carry the sharp pain and the C fibers the dull persistent pain.)

The Gate Theory of Pain

A theory of pain that accounted for all the observations, the "gate theory," was proposed by Professor Ronald Melzack of Montreal and Professor Patrick Wall of London in 1965. Melzack and Wall based their theory on histological studies of structures in the spinal cord. They proposed that the information from painful stimulation traveling up the spinal cord is modulated by a gate mechanism. If the gate is open, all the information is allowed to proceed. If the gate is partly closed or shut, less or no information is allowed to pass upward to the brain.

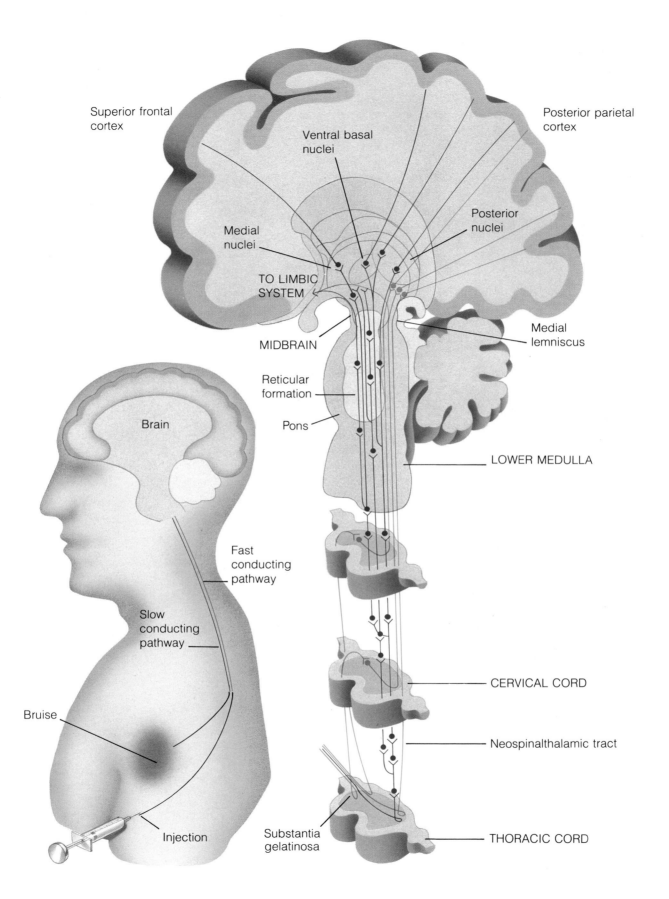

Superior frontal cortex

Posterior parietal cortex

Ventral basal nuclei

Posterior nuclei

Medial nuclei

TO LIMBIC SYSTEM

Medial lemniscus

MIDBRAIN

Reticular formation

Pons

LOWER MEDULLA

Brain

Fast conducting pathway

Slow conducting pathway

Bruise

Injection

CERVICAL CORD

Neospinalthalamic tract

Substantia gelatinosa

THORACIC CORD

The difference between slight pain and sharp pain depends on "gates" which control the passage of nerve impulses to the spinal cord (and thence to the brain). The passage of pain information from afferent fibers to spinal cord transmission (T) cells is modulated by the cells of the substantia gelatinosa (SG), which act as the spinal gating mechanism. Mild stimulation activates the large fibers, partly closing the gate and limiting the pain-information output of the T cells. A more painful stimulus increases small-fiber activity until it overcomes that in the large fibers, opening the gate and admitting more pain information.

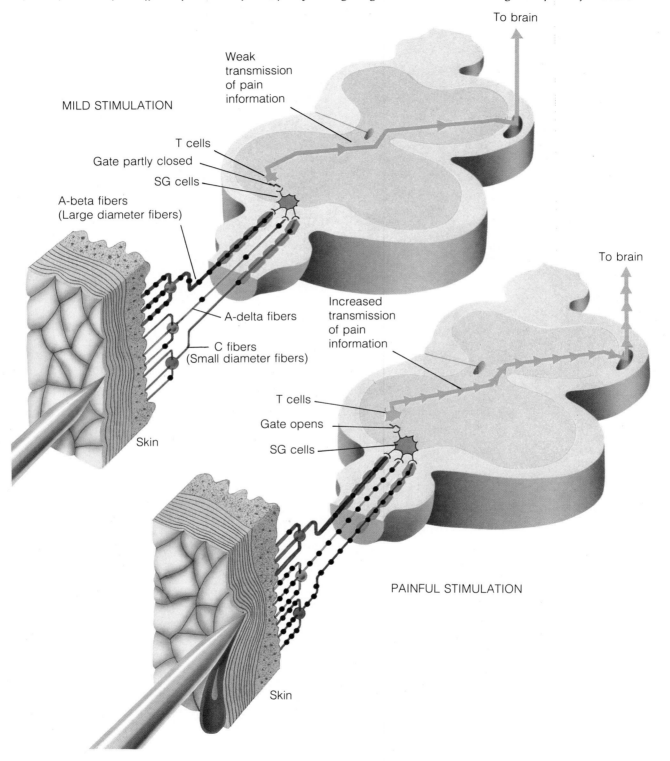

To brain

Weak
transmission
of pain
information

MILD STIMULATION

T cells

Gate partly closed

SG cells

A-beta fibers
(Large diameter fibers)

A-delta fibers

C fibers
(Small diameter fibers)

Skin

To brain

Increased
transmission
of pain
information

T cells

Gate opens

SG cells

PAINFUL STIMULATION

Skin

138

Pain information is transmitted upward by the transmission or T cell, and this cell can be activated by large or small fibers. Another cell in the substantia gelatinosa, the SG cell, has an inhibitory effect on T cell transmission. Altogether in the spinal cord there are many millions of T and SG cells. The SG cell is activated by large fiber input into the spinal cord. The C fibers, the small pain fibers, exert an inhibitory effect on the SG cells, and when no pain is felt, the fibers concerned with the perception of touch and position and the SG cell are activated. This prevents transmission from the T cell and the gate closes.

The small C fibers maintain a low level of activity in the absence of painful stimulation and hold the system in readiness for when harmful stimulation requires the gate to be opened. When a painful stimulus occurs, the small C fiber activity is increased until the total C fiber activity overcomes the inhibitory effect of the large fiber activity on the SG cell. When this happens, the SG cell ceases to hold back transmission via the T cell, and the painful stimulus travels upward.

An important balance remains between the large and small fiber systems in the perception of pain. Rubbing a painful area can make the area seem less sore. This is because the person is voluntarily increasing touch sensation, augmenting large fiber activity, inhibiting the SG cell and thus closing the gate.

In many situations, activity in the central nervous system can (sometimes voluntarily) influence the gate, either by closing it or facilitating transmission upward. If a soldier is wounded, he may feel no pain until he is removed from the battlefield. Pain perception can be suppressed through other circumstances, such as hypnosis. These are all examples of activity from higher centers closing the gate. Parts of the theory remain controversial.

Painkillers

Recently, researchers have gained a deeper understanding of pain perception as a result of studies into the receptors and neurotransmitters involved in pain pathways.

One of the earliest forms of analgesic was the drug opium, popular even before the time of the ancient Greeks from whose language is derived its

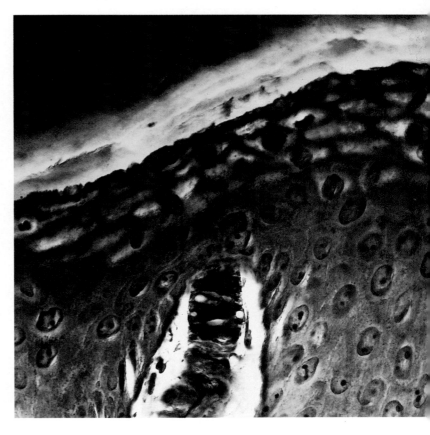

Egg-shaped Meissner's corpuscles lie just beneath the epidermis of the skin. Encapsulating sensory nerve endings, Meissner's corpuscles are believed to be touch receptors; they are most abundant in hairless skin.

English name. However, it was not until the 1850s that morphine, the pure, most active alkaloid of opium, was isolated. Since then pharmacologists have developed many compounds which have pain-relieving properties. All the most potent pain-relieving drugs, called opioids because they have the same effect as opium, have similar chemical characteristics and structural composition. (At the same time, there are other drugs with similar characteristics and composition that are not effective as analgesics.)

A factor which tends to confirm that opioids operate at a specific site of action is that opioid molecules can be easily modified to produce antagonists. An antagonist is a drug that works against another compound and reverses its effect. A simple chemical change produces nalorphine, for example, which antagonizes the analgesic effects of morphine. That such a small molecular change produces an antagonist suggests that both drugs

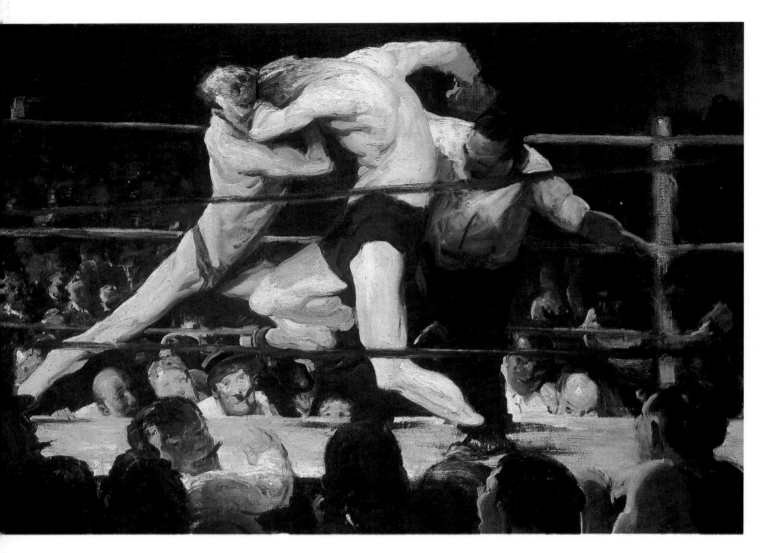

are acting at the same receptor site, and that the inhibitor prevents the analgesic molecule from binding at this site.

In 1973, Solomon Snyder and his colleagues, using drugs labeled with a radioactive material, defined the sites where opioid receptors were present, and established conclusively that these receptors did in fact exist. They were also able to show that the receptors were located near synapses and existed in the dorsal horn of the spinal cord. Opioid receptors are present in all vertebrates but absent in invertebrates.

The presence of receptors in the nervous system for morphine and related compounds suggested strongly to physiologists that the body must also have its own opioid substances for these receptors. In 1975 two small peptides were discovered which are active at the opioid receptor: these are the enkephalins. They are quickly broken down in the body, but they have now been synthesized in the

laboratory, and their effects and side effects have been shown to be the same as those of morphine; they produce analgesia, nausea, decrease respiration and alter mood. The actions of the enkephalins are opposed by the opioid antagonists that inhibit morphine. They are therefore active at the opioid receptor and are found throughout the body wherever opioid receptors are.

Another series of compounds has been found which also are active at the opioid receptor; these are called the endorphins. They are larger molecules than the enkephalins and last longer in the body. Endorphins are found in the thalamus and other parts of the brain, but not in the spinal cord. The pharmacological properties of the endorphins are also similar to those of the drugs derived from opium. They have the power to relieve pain and to reduce breathing; they alter the mood of the subject; and they have effects similar to those of the opioids on the gastrointestinal system.

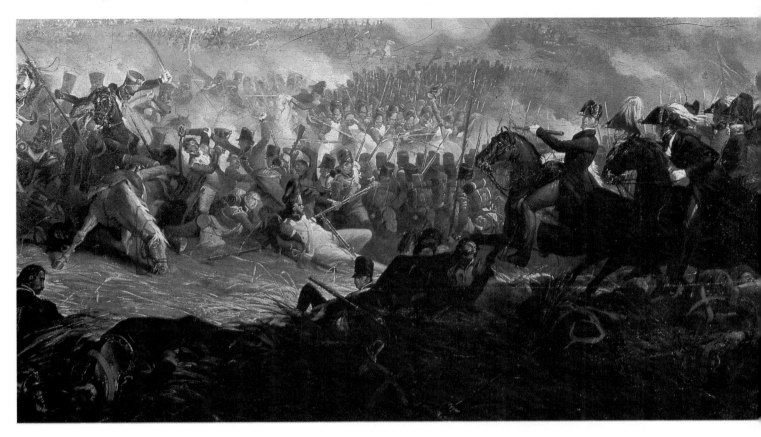

The actions of the endorphins, like those of the enkephalins, are opposed by the same group of drugs which antagonize the actions of the opioids.

As research progresses, it is becoming apparent that the opioid receptor system is more complicated than was first imagined. The enkephalins are most likely to be the neurotransmitters involved with pain perception. The endorphins have other actions. For instance, it appears that endorphins are involved in the release of some of the pituitary hormones such as growth hormone and prolactin.

Other neurotransmitters are involved in the perception of pain. It is probable that the neurotransmitter for the C fibers is substance P. The name derives from the fact that it is a powder and has no significance relating to the pain system. (In fact, it was isolated from the intestines and brains of horses in 1931.) Substance P is distributed in the C fibers of sensory nerves and in the substantia gelatinosa of the spinal cord, where it has a distribution similar to the enkephalin-containing neurons. Enkephalinlike substances and opioid analgesics inhibit the release of substance P and block pain transmission.

The integration of the nervous pathways and the chemical neurotransmitters into a coherent picture is difficult. Following a painful stimulus, a message enters the spinal cord, the dorsal horn neurons are stimulated, and the release of substance P occurs. The message of "pain" passes up the spinal cord to the brain. There are, however, neurons with enkephalins as their transmitters which inhibit pain transmission and tend to keep the gate closed.

Another group of drugs, related to acetylsalicylic acid (aspirin), acts to relieve pain in a manner completely different from the opioids. The history of aspirin really begins with the Reverend Edward Stone of Chipping Norton in England who in the late 1750s tasted the bark of a willow tree (*Salix alba*). It is probable that he did this because the barks of

Northern Thai tribeswomen cut the unripe seed pods of opium poppies. The sticky white juice from inside the pods is collected and dried to produce opium, a powerful painkilling drug. Opium and its derivatives are effective in the treatment of pain because they occupy the same sites in the brain as the body's own natural pain-relieving chemicals — the endorphins. Opium also possesses potentially dangerous addictive properties. French opium addicts (bottom) languish in the euphoric effects of the drug which occur as a result of the depressive effect of the drug on the brain and other parts of the central nervous system.

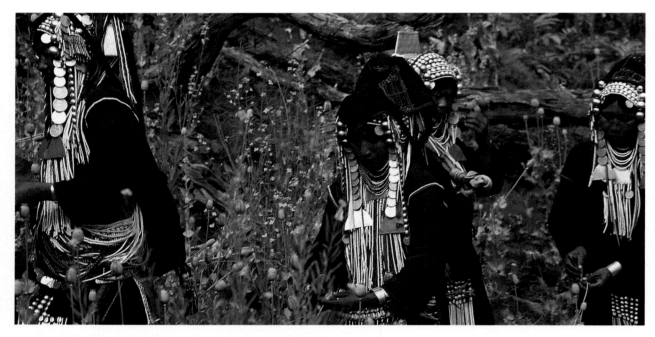

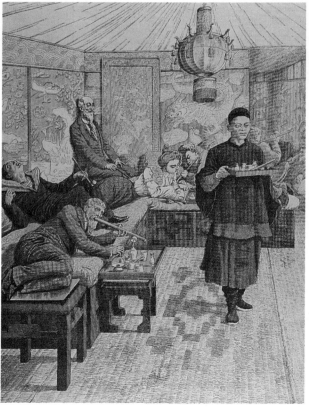

several trees were already known to have medicinal properties; the bark of the South American cinchona tree, for example, was in standard use for its action in reducing fever. Stone was encouraged to find that the willow, like the cinchona, tasted bitter. Responsible in some measure for his parishioners' temporal well-being as well as their spiritual, Stone then administered powdered willow bark to some who suffered from the ague (rigors). Altogether he treated some fifty people with the bark, and wrote to the Royal Society in 1763 about his observations of the effects.

Over the ensuing years, other scientists realized that other plants contained substances useful in treating fevers and rheumatism. In 1835, a German chemist Karl Jacob Lowig obtained an acid he called *Spirsaure* (salicylic acid). This compound was of great interest, but was very unpleasant to take and had vicious side effects. It tended to damage the mucous membranes of the digestive tract and produced pain and bleeding. Once these debilitating side effects of salicylic acid became known, only the most excruciating rheumatic condition would induce patients to take it.

Sixty years later Felix Hoffman, a chemist who worked for the Bayer company, experimented with

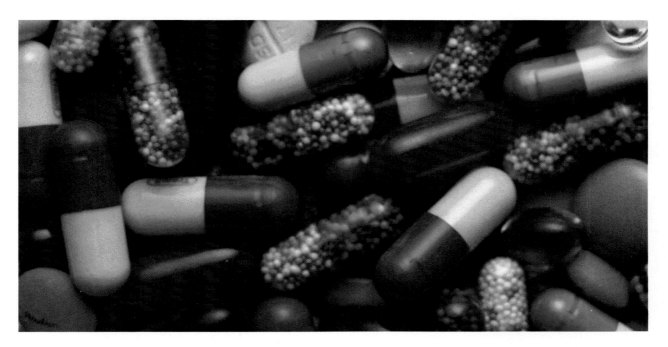

the acetylated form of salicylic acid. His main intention was to try to find a way to reduce the gastric irritant effects of sodium salicylate on behalf of his father, who was crippled with arthritis. His new formulation tasted considerably better and additionally caused fewer side effects; the name aspirin was coined for it — "a" for acetyl, and "spir" for the spiraea plant from which salicylic acid was produced.

It was not until 1971 that the mode of action of aspirin and related compounds was finally discovered. Chemical substances such as histamine are released at the site of painful stimulation. It is these pain-producing substances which stimulate electrical activity in the C fibers and initiate transmission to the brain. There are also extrinsic pain-producing substances, the two most important of which are kallikin and bradykinin. They can produce pain directly and increase sensitivity to tissue damage. These effects are increased by a group of substances, the prostaglandins, which are also produced when tissue is damaged.

Prostaglandins are long-chain fatty acids, first isolated in 1934 from seminal fluid. It was originally believed that the prostate gland was responsible for the production of these substances, hence their name. It turned out, however, that prostaglandins occur throughout the body and that there are various different compounds in the group. All are derived from a chemical called arachidonic acid, although not all are involved in pain production.

The final unraveling of the aspirin story came from work carried out by Dr John Vane at the Royal College of Surgeons in England in 1971. He showed that aspirin, and other drugs used in the treatment of inflammations (such as phenylbutazone and indomethacin), inhibited the action of the enzyme which converted arachidonic acid to prostaglandins. Arachidonic acid metabolites acting in the brain also produce fever, and this explains the effectiveness of aspirin and the other antipyretic (fever-reducing) agents. The fact that prostaglandins are produced from arachidonic acid also helps us to understand the actions of another group of drugs in the treatment of painful inflammatory conditions — the adrenocorticosteroids. Steroids act by inhibiting the production of arachidonic acid and thereby stop the pain at another stage.

Measuring Pain

One of the problems bedeviling the scientific study of pain in humans is the difficulty of measuring

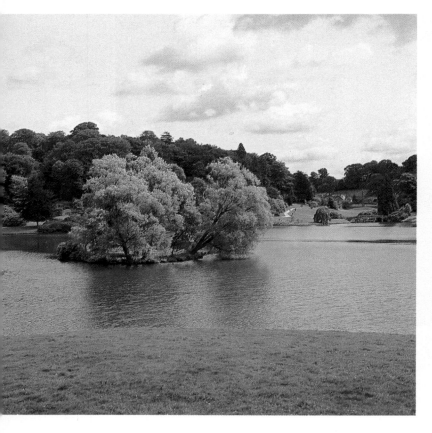

Bark from willows (below) contains salicylic acid, once used as a mild painkiller. This acid is the starting material for making aspirin (acetylsalicylic acid), although it is now produced synthetically.

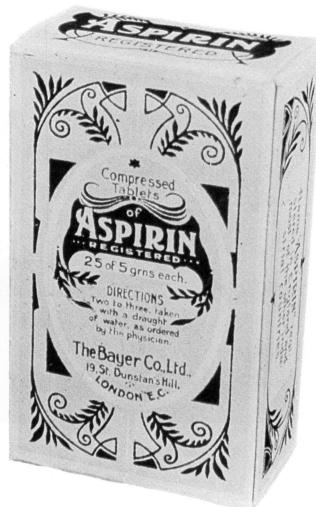

pain. Scientists and physicians like things they can quantify — quantifying pain would make it easier to compare treatments. However, things are not that easy. Everyone has a different perception of a painful stimulus, and a different threshold for feeling pain. Furthermore, perception of pain depends on the circumstances.

Similar types of painful stimuli have been used in human subjects in order to define the pain perception threshold, the point at which a stimulus (such as heat) first becomes painful, and the severe pain threshold, when the pain becomes unbearable. It has been found that although the pain perception threshold does not vary much among different socioeconomic and racial groups, there are marked variations in the severe pain threshold. It is lower, for example, among sedentary office workers than in those engaged in heavy manual labor. Thresholds are also lower in people who are depressed or over-anxious. In particularly anxious

individuals minor tranquilizers increase the threshold to pain. An interesting change in pain perception can occur when patients are given a pharmacologically inert (that is, fake) tablet or injection, known as a placebo. If the physician leads the patient to believe that the preparation is an active compound, then a placebo relieves pain in about one-third of subjects to whom it is administered.

It is unwise for a physician to try to assess someone else's pain; inevitably a marked degree of observer bias occurs. Far less subjective assessments of pain are obtained through visual linear analogue pain scales. This involves a patient being presented with a piece of paper on which there is a line 10 centimeters long. At one end is marked "I do not feel any pain" and at the other end "My pain is the worst imaginable." The patient then marks on the line where his or her current pain appears, and repeated completion of such pain scales provides

144

the physician with one of the best objective assessments of pain.

Types of Pain and Treatment

Pain occurs under many circumstances. Individuals suffer the acute pain of trauma, or the pain that occurs after surgery. There is the pain of disorders affecting muscles and bone, such as rheumatoid arthritis or a ruptured intervertebral disk. There are extremely specific pains, which are amenable to their own specific methods of treatment, such as the pain of migraine or angina. There is also the most soul-destroying of all pain, that associated with cancer.

Every physician has to evaluate each patient's pain and to plan treatment appropriately. In many centers there are pain relief clinics, often multidisciplinary, staffed by physicians from several different specialties. There may be anesthesiologists, skilled in blocking nerve transmission in various parts of the body; psychiatrists, who can help to treat the psychological aspects of pain; and neurosurgeons, who can undertake operative procedures should they be required, including nerve section (cutting) and implantation of nerve stimulators. Not all the treatments offered in a pain clinic are necessarily derived from mainstream medicine, and acupuncture or other methods of complementary medicine may also be available.

Treatment of acute postoperative pain tends to be neglected by medical and nursing staff. Pain relief after surgery is often prescribed only on a four-hourly basis, yet there have been advances in the field of postoperative pain relief. On-demand analgesia machines are now available. To use one of these, a patient presses a button and a small dose of a powerful analgesic is injected into the intravenous drip. This can be repeated as often as the patient requires — there are failsafe devices built in to these machines so that an overdose cannot be administered — but they are not without their problems. They demand a reasonably cooperative patient (capable of understanding and operating the button), a high degree of nursing maintenance — and they are expensive.

In the pain clinic, more time is available for examination and assessment of the patient and the pain. If there is no apparent physical explanation

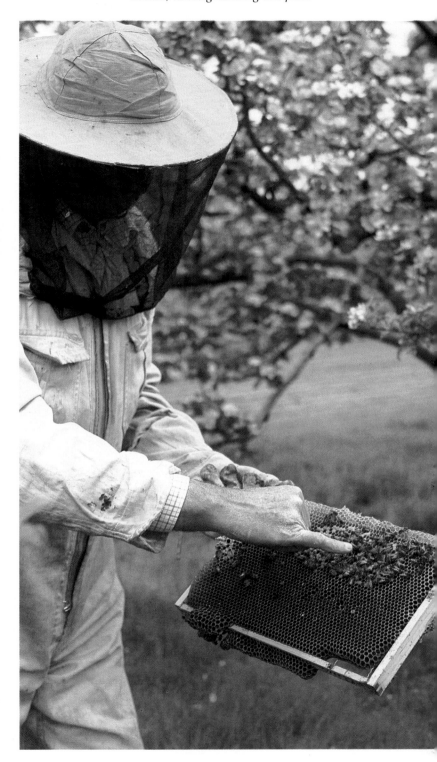

145

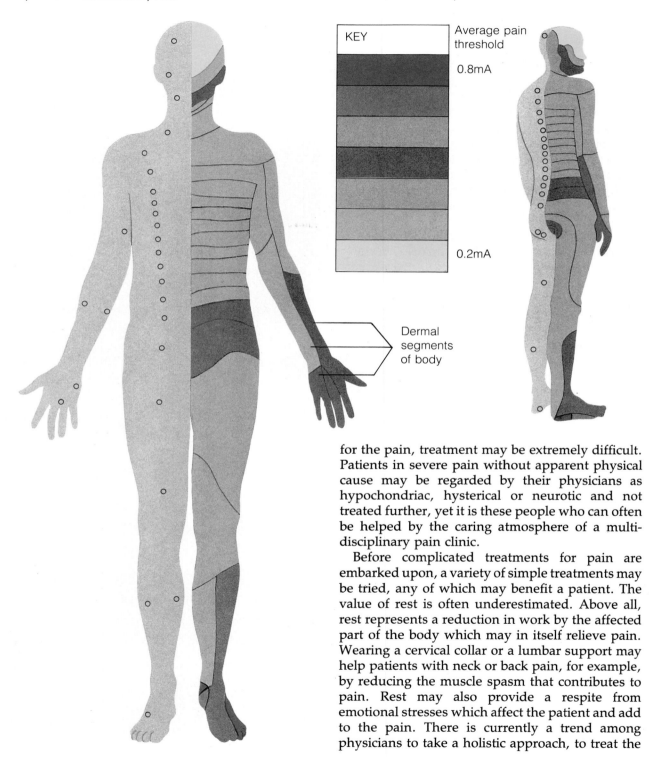

The pain threshold in the same individual is found to be fairly uniform over the entire body surface, varying with such factors as age and fatigue. Small circles indicate experimental stimulation points.

A person's pain threshold is affected by the physical demands being made on the individual. Continuous exposure to tough hard labor, with everyday minor injuries, raises the pain threshold.

KEY

Average pain threshold

0.8mA

0.2mA

Dermal segments of body

for the pain, treatment may be extremely difficult. Patients in severe pain without apparent physical cause may be regarded by their physicians as hypochondriac, hysterical or neurotic and not treated further, yet it is these people who can often be helped by the caring atmosphere of a multi-disciplinary pain clinic.

Before complicated treatments for pain are embarked upon, a variety of simple treatments may be tried, any of which may benefit a patient. The value of rest is often underestimated. Above all, rest represents a reduction in work by the affected part of the body which may in itself relieve pain. Wearing a cervical collar or a lumbar support may help patients with neck or back pain, for example, by reducing the muscle spasm that contributes to pain. Rest may also provide a respite from emotional stresses which affect the patient and add to the pain. There is currently a trend among physicians to take a holistic approach, to treat the

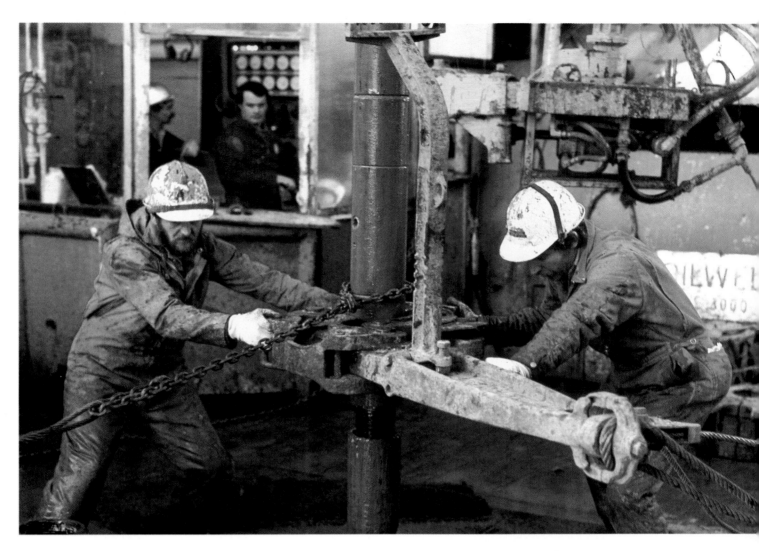

patient as a whole being, and to take into account all the circumstances rather than to treat diseases or pains in isolation.

Heat treatment has long been established as a useful method of relieving pain. Local application of heat may be employed, or other devices which supply infrared heat. Heat is effective in three ways. Firstly, heat opens up blood vessels supplying the affected area, increasing the amount of blood flowing through and helping to remove substances that produce pain locally. Secondly, heat treatment may "close the gate," may activate the SG cell and inhibit transmission from the T cell. Thirdly, heat application is both comforting and relaxing and leads to a reduction in any stresses that the patient may feel. Liniments and oils massaged into the affected area act in a similar way to heat treatment. The oils act mainly as lubricants, and the massage stimulates large fiber activity and increases blood flow.

The mainstay of any treatment of chronic pain is the use of analgesic drugs, particularly the derivatives of opium. The English physician Dr Thomas Sydenham, who lived and worked in the seventeenth century, is regarded by some as the father of clinical medicine; his book on fever (published in 1666) became a standard textbook for two centuries. In it he declared "Among the remedies which it has pleased the Almighty God to give man to relieve his sufferings none is so universal and so efficacious as opium." In addition it was Sydenham who was responsible for the introduction of a preparation of opium dissolved in alcohol, tincture of opium, or laudanum. Although a blessing as a pain-relieving medication, laudanum was freely available and caused much misery and suffering through addiction.

A semi-synthetic derivative of morphine, diacetyl morphine or heroin, appears to be more powerful than morphine, from which it is derived

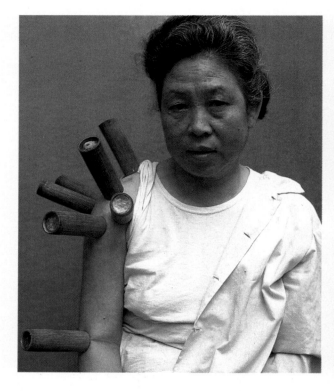

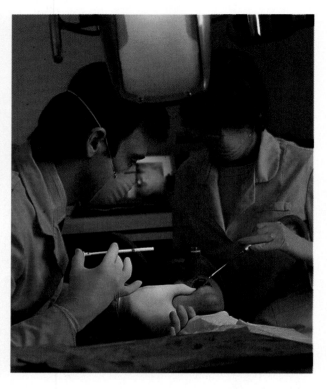

by a simple chemical process. The analgesic effect of heroin appears very quickly and produces marked euphoria. Its medical use is strictly controlled in some countries; in others, including the United States, its use is prohibited by law. The pharmaceutical industry has introduced various compounds in an attempt to provide a strong analgesic without the addictive properties of morphine, but none has replaced it. Of the less potent analgesics the most commonly used apart from aspirin is acetaminophen which, unlike aspirin, has no irritant effect on the lining of the gastrointestinal tract. It is generally regarded as of nearly equal potency with aspirin.

Another group of compounds used in the treatment of pain are the psychotropic drugs which affect the emotional state through action on the brain. They are ordinarily used in combination with analgesics and include the minor tranquilizers, such as diazepam (Valium) and the tricyclic antidepressant group of drugs. Occasionally, the major tranquilizers (for example, chlorpromazine, Thorazine) may be used. These drugs can make

pain easier to bear by reducing anxiety or lifting a depression but do not, in themselves, have any effect on the pain itself.

Sometimes analgesic therapy can produce intolerable side effects, or may not provide satisfactory pain relief even taken in the maximum dose. Under certain circumstances, especially when pain is restricted to a well-defined area, local analgesics or nerve block therapy may be effective. Local analgesic agents such as lidocaine (lignocaine) are used to treat "trigger spots," where injections are made into painful areas of muscle. Lidocaine is also used to numb areas of the body prior, for example, to dental procedures.

It is interesting that when used to treat chronic pain, the duration of relief with lidocaine is often longer than might be expected from the duration of action of the drug. This is because the freedom from pain may allow less restricted movement of a painful area and reduce any muscle spasm that may be present. A vicious pain cycle may thus be broken, in which pain leads to muscle spasm, which leads to more pain, and so on.

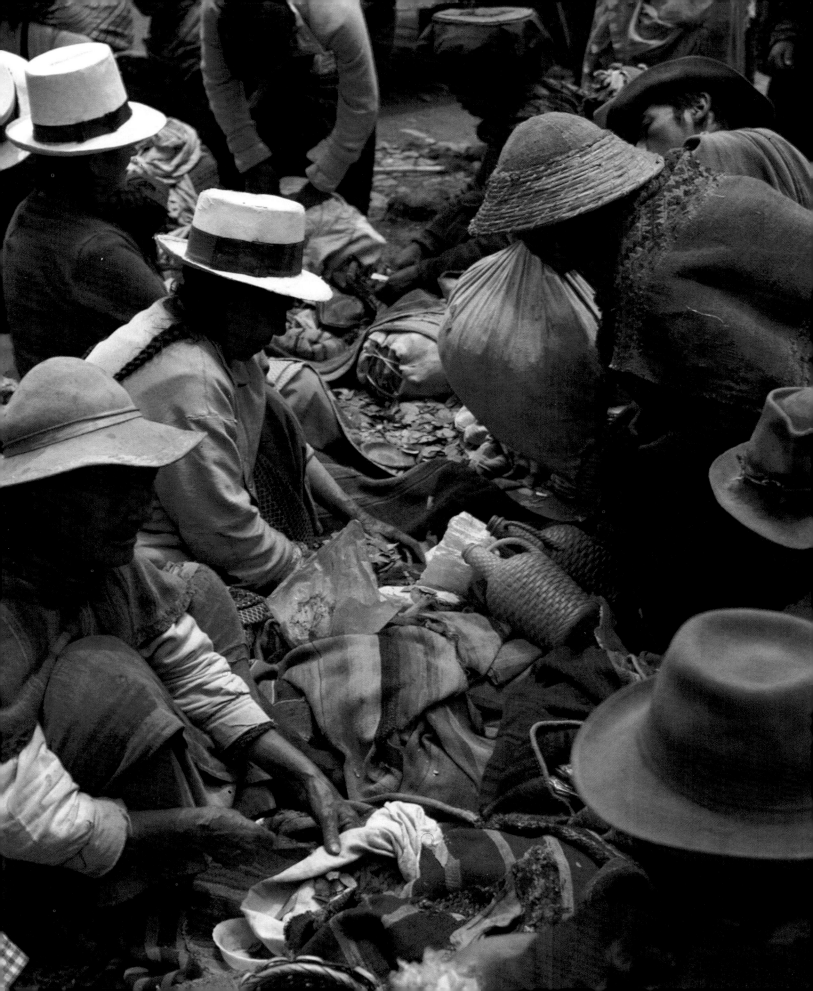

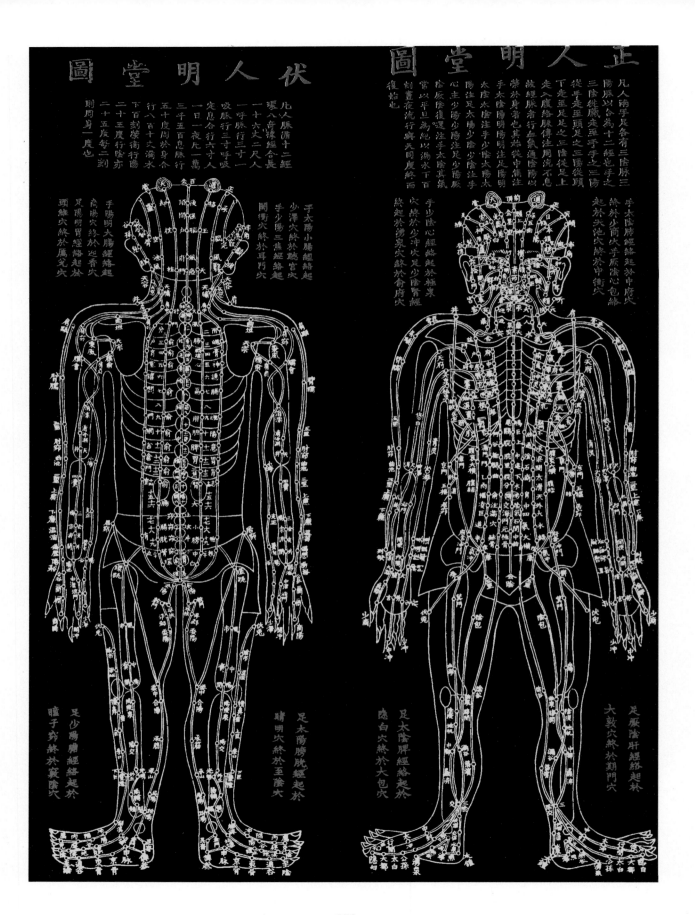

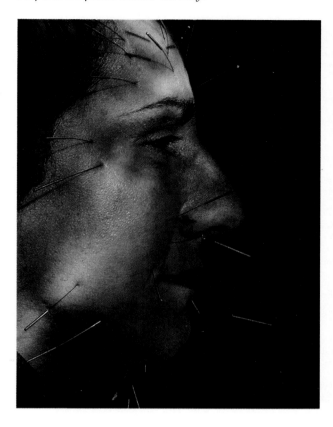

This course of action is only beneficial, however, if the freedom of movement granted is not then practiced to excess. In the late 1960s, for example, there was considerable illicit use through local injections of the steroid compound cortisone by athletes seeking to "break the pain barrier," to be able to push their bodies to the limits, and farther, without finding it too painful. The result was that several athletes permanently damaged their muscles — and at the time didn't feel a thing. Yet pain prevention — as much as pain relief — remains an important function of local anesthetics.

It is also possible to block specific nerves to treat a pain restricted to an area supplied by one or a few specific sensory nerves. Treatment may be temporary, using lidocaine, or permanent, using a neurolytic agent which destroys nerves. Two commonly used neurolytics are phenol and absolute alcohol, both of which destroy nerves if injected around them. Precise placement of the neurolytic solution must be achieved if unwanted side effects are to be avoided. It is not only sensory nerves which are blocked using such techniques. The sympathetic ganglia may also be blocked in cases of ischemic pain. When the pain is caused by poor blood supply, destroying the sympathetic nerves increases the blood supply to the limb that has been affected.

Surgical relief of pain may involve the cutting of a nerve supplying the painful area. This usually involves some sensory loss and possibly some motor loss, because most nerves are mixed. The dorsal nerve roots are only sensory, however, and may be cut if the area involved in the pain is related to only a few roots. This operation is called dorsal rhizotomy. An alternative operative procedure is antero-lateral cordotomy, in which the anterior columns of the spinal cord are cut. This can be carried out as an operative procedure under direct vision or through the skin, where a probe may be inserted which destroys the nerves by freezing.

Another method of pain relief, based on an understanding of the gate theory, is trans-cutaneous neural stimulation (TNS). This is a modification of the "rub a pain to make it better" technique. Stimulating electrodes are placed over the painful area and a mild electric current applied, producing a sensation of tingling or warmth, and may relieve pain by increasing large fiber activity and closing the gate. TNS devices are so small that they can be worn on a belt. If they are effective, they may eliminate or very much reduce the need for analgesic drugs.

An alternative, more invasive, technique is to implant the electrodes directly onto the dorsal columns of the spinal cord and stimulate the large fibers involved in the modulation of pain. This involves major surgery to attach the electrodes to the dura mater; the electrodes are activated by an external stimulator.

Although such techniques are not without risks, when effective they can transform the life of a patient plagued by chronic pain. Another method of pain treatment, now increasingly uncommon, is destruction of the pituitary gland. This is used particularly to treat pain arising from cancer which has spread to bone. The pituitary gland is situated at the base of the brain, behind the nose. Exactly how its destruction relieves pain is not understood.

Glossary

A delta fiber a type of nerve fiber with a narrow diameter and slow speed of conduction, concerned in pain transmission.

acetylcholine a chemical transmitter released at nerve endings or neuromuscular junctions.

acetylsalicylic acid a painkilling chemical, more widely known as aspirin.

adaptation the diminution of response of a nervous tissue to constant or repetitive stimuli.

adrenal medulla the central part of the adrenal, or epinephric, gland, which can be regarded as modified nerve tissue.

adrenalin a less common word for epinephrine.

adrenergic describes nerves, such as those of the sympathetic system, that release norepinephrine as a neurotransmitter.

afferent describes nerves that convey impulses from the periphery toward the central nervous system.

amino acids amine derivatives of carboxylic acids, which are the basic constituents of peptides and proteins.

analgesic with a painkilling effect.

anterior horn that part of the spinal cord where the motor nerves exit, drawn into a forward-facing "horn".

antagonize the effect of one chemical in the body on another: to oppose, inhibit or completely nullify.

antipyretic with the effect of reducing fever.

arachidonic acid a chemical from which are derived the prostaglandins, many of which are involved in producing the sensation of pain.

autoimmune disease a disease in which the body reacts against its own substances, treating them as if they were foreign.

autonomic used to describe the parts of the nervous system, the sympathetic and parasympathetic, that work largely "automatically," without conscious control.

axon the highly elongated process of a nerve cell which conducts the nerve impulse.

axonal transport the method by which substances are passed down an axon as if on a conveyor belt.

baroreceptors sense organs that react to changes in pressure.

bouton enlargement at the synapse end of the tiny, branched terminal of an axon.

brachial in the arm region.

bradykinin one of a group of biochemical substances capable of producing pain.

C fiber a non-myelinated nerve fiber, of small diameter, which can transmit pain stimuli.

causalgia an intense burning sensation experienced following some types of nerve damage.

cephalization the evolutionary tendency to concentrate nervous tissue and major sense organs at the "head".

cerebellum a posterior lobe of the brain behind the entry of the spinal cord and beneath the hemispheres; its main function is the coordination of the muscles concerned in body movements.

cervical of the neck.

cholinergic describes nerves which use acetylcholine as a neurotransmitter.

cholinesterase an enzyme that breaks down acetylcholine.

coccygeal of the coccyx, the fused bones at the lower end of the spine.

conductance the capacity for conveying a neural (electrical) impulse.

cordotomy surgical cutting of part of the spinal cord.

cortex the surface or outer layer of an organ, as opposed to the inner medulla.

cranial nerve a nerve arising from the central nervous system within the skull.

dendrite one of many short processes which can receive impulses and conduct them to the nerve cell body.

depolarized describes a nerve cell in which the normal polarization of the membrane, the interior negative to the exterior, has been disturbed or has disappeared, usually in conjunction with the passage of a nerve impulse.

dermatome an area of skin innervated by one spinal nerve, corresponding to one embryonic segment.

dorsal root the dorsal half of the "forked" configuration of each spinal nerve as it connects with the spinal cord; sensory nerves from the periphery enter the cord along this root.

efferent describes nerves which convey impulses away from the central nervous system.

electrophysiology techniques which use, record and measure electrical phenomena to find out more about the workings of the body.

end plate the area on a muscle fiber where the fine branches of a motor nerve fiber come to an end, by which the muscle can be excited into action.

endocrine describes glands, or their secretions, where secretion takes place directly into the bloodstream rather than by ducts.

endorphin a body substance that may be of importance in pain control, and in the release of some hormones.

enkephalin a body substance thought to act as a neurotransmitter in the modification of pain perception.

epinephrine a hormone produced by the adrenal medulla, a powerful stimulator of the sympathetic nervous system.

euphoria a sense of well-being, contentment; in psychiatry it suggests a state that may not be consistent with external circumstances.

exocrine describes glands from which secretion takes place through ducts.

facilitating diminishing or eliminating a nerve's resistance to subsequent stimulation.

foramen an opening, especially through or into a bone (or tooth).

ganglion a "knot" or group of neurons, generally of those of the peripheral nervous system; sometimes, however, the term refers to specific groups of nerve cells in the brain or spinal cord.

gate theory a theory of pain perception that supposes that onward transmission of pain messages is allowed or prevented by "gates" which are either open or closed, depending on the balance of opposing excitatory or inhibitory nerves.

giant axon a large nerve fiber of a type found in some mollusks such as the squid. Giant axons can be 0.5 mm in diameter, and have proved very useful subjects for experiments on the electrical phenomena of nerve impulses.

giant fiber a large nerve (in a worm, for example) that allows rapid communication through the length of the body.

glial cells neuroglia.

glucostat a physiological mechanism that allows the maintenance of a constant concentration of glucose in the blood.

glycogen a carbohydrate that acts as a storage product in animals, found especially in the liver.

gray matter parts of the spinal cord and brain in which the nerves do not have a myelin sheath and so appear grayish on gross dissection.

gyri the "hills" of the brain's outer surface which, with the sulci (the "valleys"), by their folds maximize the surface area of the brain.

hemisection cutting (an organ) in half or halfway through.

holistic with reference to the whole being; as in medical practice which considers all aspects of a person's health and lifestyle, rather than trying only to alleviate symptoms.

hormones secretions of ductless glands within the body which may affect local or distant parts of the body, or the whole body.

hypothalamus a part of the brain below the third ventricle which maintains control of many aspects of the body's internal environment.

inhibitory with the effect of tending to prevent the passage of a nerve impulse.

interneuron a nerve cell which is neither attached to a sense organ nor to an effector unit, but acts purely as a relay cell.

intervertebral disk one of the disks of cartilage between each pair of vertebrae. If injured or displaced, the disk may press on a spinal nerve and cause pain.

invertebrate any animal that does not have a backbone.

ion an atom or molecule that carries an electric charge.

limbic system a group of structures located in an arch around the front of the brainstem; the limbic system affects emotional behavior.

lumbar in or near the lower part of the back.

medulla the inner part or layer of an organ, as opposed to the outer cortex.

meninges the membranes which form an envelope around the brain and spinal cord.

microelectrode a tiny electrode used to explore electrical activity in nerves and muscles. Often it consists of a glass tube drawn out to a very fine tip which can be filled with a conducting solution and inserted within a cell.

microtubule one of the small intracellular tubules found in the cytoplasm of many cells.

modality the mode or type of a sensation or sensory stimulus.

morphine a principal alkaloid of opium, first isolated in 1806; a strong painkilling drug, it and its derivatives are in constant medical use.

morula the early embryo, when it is little more than a ball of dividing cells.

motor neurons nerve cells leading to the muscles; impulses from motor neurons initiate and regulate body movements.

myelin the refracting fatty substance that makes up much of the sheath round many nerve fibers and is responsible for their white appearance. It also helps considerably to speed up the transmission of neural impulses, although how it does so is not understood.

myotome all the muscle that corresponds to a single segment of an embryo and is basically innervated by a single segmental nerve trunk.

nerve net a type of nervous system found in some primitive animals, in which the nerve cells communicate, via synapses, with their neighbors, but in which there is no central nervous system or major pathways.

neural crest a crest of cells on either side of the dorsal midline in an early embryo, which develops to form the ganglia of the dorsal roots of spinal nerves.

neural tube the embryonic beginnings of the central nervous system, formed by the folding of the embryonic disk.

neuroblast an embryonic cell from which nerve cells develop.

neuroblocker a disrupter of the system by which chemicals are set to travel across a synapse to transmit an impulse from one nerve to another.

neurofilament one of the microscopic intracellular filaments found especially in axons, associated with transport of materials.

neuroglia the numerous supporting cells of the nervous system in which the nerve cells are embedded.

neurolemmal sheath the collagenous sheath surrounding a nerve fiber.

neurologist a scientist who studies the anatomy and physiology of the nervous system; specialist in nervous diseases.

neurolysis the destruction of nerve tissue (often by acid); or the longitudinal cutting of the myelin sheath around a nerve.

neuropathy disease of the nerves.

neurosecretory cells cells of the nervous system which have a glandular function, such as those of the pituitary body.

neurotransmitter any substance produced at the tips of one nerve cell that is able to trigger or inhibit the start of an impulse in the next.

Nissl substance a dense aggregation of endoplasmic reticulum near the nucleus of a nerve cell.

node of Ranvier one of the gaps in the insulating myelin sheath around a nerve.

non-medullated unmyelinated; without the myelin sheath.

norepinephrine a neurotransmitter in some nerve cells, such as those of the sympathetic system; alternatively known as noradrenalin.

oligodendrocytes neuroglia which sheathe many of the longer nerve axons and contain a large number of microtubules.

opioids pain-relieving substances that have similar effects to opium.

optic chiasma the junction of the two optic nerves.

oscilloscope an instrument for recording electrical phenomena and displaying them by means of a cathode-ray tube's fluorescent screen.

osmoreceptor a sense organ monitoring the concentration of substances in the body fluids.

parasympathetic belonging to that part of the autonomic nervous system which supplies glands and smooth muscles; its nerves originate in the brain or in the sacral region, and many of its actions are broadly opposed to those of the sympathetic system.

permeability the extent to which a membrane allows the passage of a substance through it.

physiology the way in which a body functions (as distinct from its anatomy).

pituitary gland a small but vital endocrine gland in the center of the head, responsible mainly for regulation of the hormonal balance of the body.

placebo an inert substance given by a medical experimenter, without the knowledge of the patient, as a substitute for an active one, for the purpose of comparison.

plexus a network of interwoven nerves, especially one formed from the main branches of nerve trunks, such as those in the brachial, lumbar and sacral regions.

postganglionic describes autonomic nerve fibers proceding from a ganglion.

presynaptic before a synapse, for example, the terminals of an axon and their contained vesicles of neurotransmitter.

proprioceptor a sense organ that responds to stimuli from within the body, such as those that monitor the state of muscular contraction.

prostaglandins long-chain fatty acids, so named because they were originally found in prostate gland products: they seem to be involved in producing the sensation of pain.

psychotropic describes drugs that have effects on the moods and emotions.

ramus a branch.

receptor a sensory nerve cell terminal sensitive to specific types of stimuli, physical or chemical.

referred pain pain which is felt not at the site of an injury, inflammation, or disease, but in some other part of the body, the reason being that both parts are innervated by the same major segmental nerve.

reflex an action brought about by a stimulus automatically, and involuntarily, with transmission of impulses through the nervous system often not reaching the level of consciousness or reaching it only after action has been taken.

resting potential the difference in electrical potential that can be measured between the inside and the outside of a nerve cell which is not in the process of transmitting an impulse.

rhizotomy surgical cutting of the roots of spinal nerves.

sacral of or near the part of the backbone to which the hip-bones are attached.

Schwann cell one of the cells which are wrapped round and round a nerve fiber and make the myelin sheath of a nerve fiber, thus constituting "white matter" as opposed to "gray matter."

section the surgical cutting of tissue.

sensory neuron a nerve cell that conveys information from a sense organ toward the central nervous system.

sodium pump theory a hypothesis to explain the maintenance of electrical potential differences across the membranes of a nerve cell.

somatic of the body (the somatic sensory area of the brain, for example, deals with sensations from various parts of the body); also used to distinguish body cells from reproductive cells.

somite one of the divisions or segments identifiable in the body of an embryo.

spastic subject to spasm (contraction of a muscle, or constriction of a passage or orifice).

spinal cord nerve tissue contained within the vertebral canal in the backbone.

spinal nerve one of the nerve trunks that emerges from the backbone (the spine).

spinothalamic tract a nerve tract running to the thalamus from the spinal cord.

substance P a neurotransmitter in the small pain-conducting C fibers.

substantia gelatinosa the jellylike substance of the dorsal part of the spinal cord.

sulci the "valleys" of the brain's outer surface which, with the gyri (the "hills"), by their folds maximize the surface area of the brain.

summation the combined effect of the arrival of two or more nerve impulses at a synapse (temporal summation) or of the activation of two or more synapses onto the same nerve (spatial summation).

sympathetic describes the system of motor nerves supplying glands and smooth muscles, and originating in the cervical, thoracic and lumbar regions of the spinal cord. Many of its actions are antagonistic to those of the parasympathetic system.

synapse the specialized region where two nerve cells come into close contact, and across which an impulse can be transmitted, usually via the agency of transmitter substances.

synaptic cleft the small gap at a synapse between two nerve cells.

terminal bouton one of the swollen endings on the fine branch tips at the end of an axon.

thalamus part of the brain near the midline below the cerebral hemispheres to which run all the nerves that give rise to conscious sensation.

thermoreceptor a sense organ that reacts to heat stimuli.

thoracic in the region of the chest.

threshold the point up to which a stimulus has no effect, and beyond which it sets off a reaction.

thymus a ductless gland of the lower neck region which disappears by the time of adulthood.

toxoid a toxin made harmless but retaining its capacity to stimulate antibodies.

tract in neurology, a group of nerve fibers together responsible for the conveying of information concerning a specific sense.

ventral root the root of a spinal nerve emerging forward and downward, containing motor fibers.

vesicle a small sac, such as the ones that hold neurotransmitter at the tips of nerves.

white matter part of the brain or spinal cord consisting mainly of myelinated axons; it is the myelination that in fact makes up the visibly white part, the normal coloration of nerves being the gray hue that is generally described in gray matter.

Illustration Credits

Introduction
Synaptek Scientific Products
Incorporated/Science Photo Library.

Mapping the Maze
8, *Le Cirque* by G. Seurat/The Louvre,
Paris/The Bridgeman Art Library. 10,
Martin Dohrn/Science Photo Library. 11, *City Activities* by Thomas Hart
Benton/Courtesy of The Equitable.
12, Tony Stone Worldwide.
13, Royal Albert Memorial Museum,
Exeter/The Bridgeman Art Library. 14,
Borghese Gallery, Rome/SCALA. 16,
National Library of Medicine. 17,
Bodleian Library, Oxford. 18, *The Anatomy Lesson* by Rembrandt/
Mauritshuis, The Hague/The
Bridgeman Art Library. 19,
Reproduced by gracious permission of
Her Majesty, Queen Elizabeth II, 20, Ann
Ronan Picture Library. 21, *Esperimento della pila di Alessandro Volta Firenze,
Tribuna di Galileo*, Museo Zoologica,
"La Specola"/SCALA. 22, Ann Ronan
Picture Library. 23, The Mansell
Collection. 25, Manfred Kage/Science
Photo Library.

Simplicity to Sophistication
26, Tony Stone Worldwide. 28, Frank
Whitney/The Image Bank. 29, The
Mansell Collection. 30, (top) Georges
Tourdjman/The Image Bank, (bottom)
Marshal Sklar/Science Photo Library.
31, Biophoto Associates. 32, Tony
Stone Worldwide. 33, Peter Newark's
Western Americana. 34, **Aziz Khan**.
35, Tony Stone Worldwide. 36, Bill
Wood/Seaphot Ltd: Planet Earth
Pictures. 37, Tony Stone Worldwide.
38, Peter David/Seaphot Ltd: Planet
Earth Pictures. 39, (left) Mike Coltman/
Seaphot Ltd: Planet Earth Pictures,
(right) Walter Deas/Seaphot Ltd: Planet
Earth Pictures. 40, **Mick Gillah**. 41,
Carl Roessler/Seaphot Ltd: Planet Earth
Pictures.

Ionic Impulses
42, Biophoto Associates. 44, (top) **Mick
Saunders**, (bottom) Barrie Rokeach/The
Image Bank. 45, *Horizontal Tree* by Piet
Mondrian/Munson-Williams-Procter
Institute, Utica, New York. 46, The
Mansell Collection. 47, (left) **Mick
Gillah**, (right) Biophoto Associates. 48,
David Parker/Science Photo Library.
49, (top) London Fire Brigade, (bottom)
Aziz Khan. 50, (top) **Mick Saunders**,
(bottom) Harald Sind/The Image Bank.
51, David Redfern. 52, (top) Godfrey
Argent, (bottom) Godfrey Argent. 53,
The Photosource. 54, Biophoto
Associates. 55, Tony Stone Worldwide.
56, Tony Stone Worldwide. 57, (top)
Tony Stone Worldwide, (bottom) Gene
Cox/Science Photo Library. 58, **Aziz
Khan**. 59, BBC Hulton Picture Library.
60, The Photosource. 61, Vaughan
Fleming/Science Photo Library.

Selective Systems
62, The Mansell Collection. 64 & 65,
A.W.K.A. Popkiewicz & Susan Smith.
66, Sally and Richard Greenhill. 67,
Ann Ronan Picture Library. 69,
Aerospace Corporation/Science Photo
Library. 70, (top) Biophoto Associates,
(bottom) A. McClenaghan/Science
Photo Library. 71, (top) Mary Evans
Picture Library, (bottom) National
Library of Medicine. Foldout, (outside
A) The Mansell Collection, (outside B)
Biophoto Associates, (inside) **Mick
Gillah, Aziz Khan**, (outside C) John
Watney Photo Library, (outside D) The
Mansell Collection. 73, *The Nervous
System* by Malcolm Poynter/Nicholas
Treadwell Galleries. 74, Sally and
Richard Greenhill. 75, *The Distinguished
Visitor* by Jan Brueghel,
Kunsthistorisches Museum, Vienna/
The Bridgeman Art Library. 77, Mary
Evans Picture Library. 79, B. Rose/The
Image Bank.

Automatic Actions
80, Tony Stone Worldwide. 82, Mary
Evans Picture Library. 83, **Mick Gillah**.
85, **Mick Gillah**. 86, **Mick Gillah**. 87,
David Parker/Science Photo Library.
88, (left) Martin Dohrn/Science Photo
Library, (right) Martin Dohrn/Science
Photo Library. 89, The Fotomas Index.
91, (top) *Winter Scene* from *The Four
Seasons* by Shoun/The Bridgeman Art
Library, (bottom) Dr. R. Clark & M.
Goff/Science Photo Library. 92, Tony
Stone Worldwide. 93, Dr. R. Clark &
M. Goff/Science Photo Library. 94,
Mick Gillah. 95, Geoff du Feu/Seaphot
Ltd: Planet Earth Pictures. 96, Mary
Evans Picture Library. 97, The Mansell
Collection.

Conception to Completion
98, Tony Stone Worldwide. 100 **Mick
Saunders**. 101, (top) **Mick Saunders**,
(bottom) Camera Talks. 102, **Mick
Saunders**. 103, (top) Margaret W.
Peterson/The Image Bank, (bottom) Ulli
Seer/The Image Bank. 104, Sally and
Richard Greenhill. 105, Robert Harding
Picture Library. 106, Biophoto
Associates. 107, Tony Stone
Worldwide. 108, Dr. C. Chumbley/
Science Photo Library. 109, (top) *Try
This Pair* by F. D. Hardy/The Guildhall
Art Gallery, City of London/The
Bridgeman Art Library, (bottom) Sally
and Richard Greenhill. 110, Sally and
Richard Greenhill. 111, (top) Sally and
Richard Greenhill, (bottom) Tom
McCarthy/The Image Bank. 112, (top)
Burton McNeely/The Image Bank,
(bottom) Ulli Seer/The Image Bank.
113, ASBAH. 114, (left) ASBAH, (right)
ASBAH. 115, Sally and Richard
Greenhill.

Short Circuits in the System
116, SCALA. 118, (top) Robin Williams/
Science Photo Library, (bottom) Sally
and Richard Greenhill. 119, **Aziz
Khan**. 120, (left) Mary Evans Picture
Library, (right) Jim Stevenson/Science
Photo Library. 121, *The Madhouse* from
The Rake's Progress by Hogarth/Sir John
Soane Museum/The Bridgeman Art
Library. 122, John Watney Photo
Library. 123, **Aziz Khan**. 124, (top) Dr.
R. Clark & M. Goff/Science Photo
Library, (bottom) John Watney Photo
Library. 125, John Walsh Science Photo
Library. 126, (left) Ann Ronan Picture
Library, (right) John Watney Photo
Library. 127, (top) **Mick Gillah**,
(bottom) *Cottage Industry* by W. Hinks/
British Museum/The Bridgeman Art
Library. 128, (left) John Watney Photo
Library, (right) Sally and Richard
Greenhill. 129, The Mansell Collection.
130, The Fotomas Index. 131, Biophoto
Associates. 132, Sally and Richard
Greenhill. 133, (top) Peter Newark's
Western Americana, (left) The Imperial
War Museum.

Agony and Ecstasy
134, Robert Harding Picture Library.
137, **Mick Gillah**. 138, **Mick Gillah**.
139, Biophoto Associates. 140, *Stag at
Sharkey's* by George Wesley Bellows/
The Cleveland Museum of Art,
Hinman B. Hurlbut Collection. 141,
Battle of Waterloo by Denis Dighton/
Marquess of Anglesea/The Bridgeman
Art Library. 142, (top) J. M. Hobday/
Natural Science Photos, (bottom) Mary
Evans Picture Library. 143, Martin
Dohrn/Science Photo Library. 144, (left)
Heather Angel, (right) Bayer Co. 145,
Tony Stone Worldwide. 146, **Mick
Gillah**. 147, Tony Stone Worldwide.
148, (left) Sally and Richard Greenhill,
(right) Gary Gladstone/The Image
Bank. 149, South American Picture
Library. 150, Mary Evans Picture
Library. 151, Tony Stone Worldwide.

Index

Fallopian tube, 99
fat, 94
fatty acid, 90
feeding center, 92
fetus, 104
fever, 90, 143
fiber nerve, 47, 52, 57
  giant, 38
fight-or-flight response, 81, 97, **97**
flatworm, 38, 40
folic acid, 114
forebrain, 84, 106, 108
frontal cortex, 112

G
Galen, 15
gall bladder, 90
Galvani, Luigi, **21**, 22, 23, 24
gamma-aminobutyric acid, 61
ganglion,
  cerebral, 38, 39
  dorsal root, 68, 74, 120
  mesenteric, 87
  nerve, 16, 38, 41, 82, 84
  sympathetic, 105, 106, 151
  vertebral, 30
gastrectomy, 132
gastrointestinal tract, *see* digestive tract
genitalia, 88
glandular, 131
glaucoma, 95
gliablast, **102**
glial cell, 45, 100, 102–103
glossopharyngeal nerve, 68
glucose, 81, **87**, 90, 92, 97
glycogen, 90, 97
gray matter, 33, 48, 74, **100–101**
Guillain-Barre syndrome, 131
gut, 136
gyrus, 108

H
hair, 97, **103**
hamstring, 72
hand, 72
head, 68
heart, 23, 85, 88, 90, 94, 97, **123**, 135, 136
heartbeat, 80, 105
  abnormal, 95
Helmholtz, Hermann von, 24
hemorrhage, 90
  cerebral, 129
heroin, 147–148
Herophilus, 14
Herpes zoster, 120, **120**
hindbrain, 106
Hippocrates, 14
histamine, 143, **145**
Hodgkin, Alan, 52
hormone, 10, 35, 82, 97, 108
humerus, 72, 126

hunger, 90
Huxley, Andrew, 52
hydrocephaly, 113, **114, 115**
hydrophobia, 120
hypertension, 95, 129
hypnosis, 129, 139
hypoglossal nerve, 68, **74**
hypothalamus, 84, 90, 92, 95, 97, 106

I
insect, 39, **40**
insulin, 132
interneuron, 65
intervetebral foramen, 70
intestine, **43**, 84, **87**, 88, 97
intrinsic factor, 132
ion, 48, 49, 50, 52, 53, 60
isoproterenol, 95

J
jellyfish, 36, **40**

K
kallikin, 143
kidney, 22, 87, 88, 95, 106

L
Langley, J. N., 82
laudanum, 147
Leonardo da Vinci, **19**
leprosy, 122, 131
lidocaine, 148
limb bud, 103, **105**
limbic system, 84
lipid, 44
liver, 15, 84, **87**, 90, 94
Loewi, Otto, 59
lumbago, 125
lumbar puncture, 105
lung, 88, 95, 97, **119**
lupus erythematosus, 132
lymphocyte, 122

M
Magendie, François, 24, 68, 71
magnetic resonance imaging, 125
malformation, congenital, 113
Malpighi, Marcello, 19
measles, 122
median nerve, 72, 126, **127**
medulla, 84, 136
melanocyte, 102, **103**
Melzack, Ronald, 136
membrane, cell, 44, 46, 49, 53, 54, 57
memory, 9
meninges, 102
menopause, 10
menstruation, 10
mesencephalon, 84, 106
microelectrode, 48

microscope, electron, 12
microtubule, 45
midbrain, 84, 106, 136
migraine, 95, 145
mitochondrion, 44, **119**
mollusk, 32, 39
morphine, 139, 140
morula, 99
motor,
  end plate, 57, 59, 78
  impulse, 63, **64, 65**
  nerve, 10, 21, 24, 57, **58**, 120
  neuron disease, **128**, 129
  root, 102
mucopolysaccharide, 57
mucus, secretion of, 81
Müller, Johannes, 24, 46
multiple sclerosis, 122–124, 129
muscarine, 94
muscle, 65, 76, 94, 130
  skeletal, 81, 94, 97
  smooth, 94, **94**
muscle spindle, 65
muscular dystrophy, 128
myasthenia gravis, 130
Mycobacterium leprae, 122
myelin, 29, 32, 46, 47, **47, 54**, 57, **60**, 74, 76, 102, **102**, 122, 131, 132
myelination, 108–110
myelogram, 125
myocardial infarction, 135
myocyte, **39**
myotome, 100, 104
myotonia congenita, 128

N
nalorphine, 139
nasal gland, 88
nasopharynx, 19
neck, 68
neostigmine, 130
nerve cell, 27, 28
nerve fiber, 38, 47, 52, 57
nerve net, 36
nervous system,
  autonomic, 29, 41, 60, 63, 66, **81**, 82, **82**, 84, 90, **94**, 95, **96**, 97, **97**, 105, 136
  central, 7, 27, 29, 33, 47, 57, 61, 63, 72, 74, 78, 82, 139
  parasympathetic, 29, 30, 41, 82, **83**, 93, **94**, 97, 105, 106
  peripheral, 10, 27, 41, 47, 61, 68, 72, 74, 104, **117, 119**, 125, 130, 136
  sympathetic, 16, 19, 29, 30, **32**, 82, **83, 85**, 90, 93, **94**, 95, 105, 106, 151
neural crest, 100, 102, 105, 106
neural tube, 100, **100**, 102, 113
neuralgia, trigeminal, 125
neuroblast, 100, **100**, 102, **102**, 105
neuroepithelium, 100, 106
neurofibroma, 128
neurofibromatosis, 126

neurofilament, 45
neuroglia, 45
neuromuscular spindle, **70**
neuron, **30**, **44**, **101**, **102**
   motor, 29, 33, 76, 118, 130
   sensory, 33, **34**
neuropraxis, 125
neurosecretory cell, 35
neurotomesis, 125
neurotransmitter, 28, 82, 94, 139
neurotubule, 45
nicotine, 94
Nissl substance, 44
norepinephrine, 61, 87, **87**, 92, 93, **94**, 97
nucleus, 46, **47**, 68

O
octopus, **38**, 39
oculomotor nerve, 68
odontoblast, 102, **103**
olfactory nerve, 68
oligodendrocyte, 45, **102**
opioid, 139–140
opium, 139, **142**
optic nerve, 68, 110, 111
organelle, 28, 44, **44**
oscilloscope, 48, **48**
osmoreceptor, 92
ovary, 10
ovum, 99
oxygen, 45, 97, 135

P
pain, 135–139, **136**
   gate theory of, 136, **138**
pancreas, 132
paralysis, 12, 16, 76, 94, **119**, 125
   spastic, 65
Pasteur, Louis, 46
pelvic nerve, 88
penicillin, 121, **121**
pepsin, 46
peristalsis, 88, **123**
pernicious anemia, 132
peroneal muscular atrophy, 128
phenol, 151
phrenic nerve, 72
physostigmine, 94
pituitary gland, 32, 35, 108, 151
placenta, 104
plasma cell, 122
plasmapheresis, 131
plexus, 72
   brachial, 126
   solar, 105
poliomyelitis, 118, **118**, **119**
polyarteritis nodosa, 131
polyneuropathy, 132
pons, 106
postganglionic nerve, 88, 93, 94
postsynaptic region, 57
potassium, 44, 48, **49**, 50, 51, 52, 59, 60

potassium channel, 60
potential,
   end-plate, 59
   resting, 48, 51
Pott's disease, 125
preganglionic nerve, 88, 93, **94**
premedication, **96**
presynaptic region, 57
proprioreceptors, 63, 76, **79**
prostaglandin, 143
protein, 44, 54
primitive groove, **100**
prosencephalon, 106
puberty, 10
pupil, 88, **88**, 106

R
rabies, 118–120, **120**
radial nerve, 72
ramus, gray, 105
Ranvier, nodes of, 47, 57
receptor,
   norepinephrine, 94, 95
   sensory, **29**, **39**, 74
rectum, 88
reflex,
   grasping, 111
   pupillary, 21
   rooting, 111
   spinal, 64–65
   sucking, 110
   swimming, 110–111
reflex arc, 32, 33, **34**, 64, **67**, 84, **85**
reflex loop, 21
respiration, 81
respiratory tract, **96**
retina, 95
rhizotomy, dorsal, 151
rhombencephalon, 106
Richet, Charles, 82

S
Sabin, Albert, 118
sacrum, 104
salbutamol, 95
saliva, **87**, **88**
salivary gland, 88, **88**, 106
Salk, Jonas, 118
satiety center, 92
Schwann, Theodor, 45, 46
Schwann cell, 45–47, **47**, 102, **102**, 103
sciatica, 125
sciatic nerve, 72
sea anemone, 36, 38, **39**
sea cucumber, 41
sea squirt, 41
sea urchin, 41, **41**
sensory cell, 41
sensory impulse, 63, **64**, 65
sensory nerve, 15, 19, 24, 29
sensory root, 102
sexual response, 90
SG-cell, 139

sheath, glial, 47
shingles, 120, **120**
shivering, 90
skin, 14, 21, 102, **103**, **120**
skull, 108, 125
slow virus, 122
smooth muscle, 94, **94**
sodium, 48, 49, **49**, 50, **50**, 51, 53, 59, 60
sodium channel, 54, 57, 60
sodium chloride, 44, 48
sodium-potassium pump, **49**, 51–54
somite, 100, 104
sperm, 99
spider, 39
spina bifida, 113, **113**, **115**
spinal cord, 9, 14, 16, 21, 32, 33, 41, 47, 61, 63, 64, 65, 66, 68, 70, 74, 76, 84, **85**, 87, 88, 95, 100, **101**, 102, 106, 112, 113, 115, 117, 118, 120, **124**, 130, 136, 139, 151
spinal nerve, 68, 100, 102, 104, 106, 125
spine, 27, 29, **34**
spine, dendritic, 43
spinothalamic tract, 74, 136
spleen, 97
spondylosis, cervical, 125
sponge, 36, **39**, **40**
squid, 39, 43, 52
starfish, 41
steroid, 124, 128
stomach, 68, 84, 87, 88
strychnine, 66, 71
substance-P, 141
substantia gelatinosa, 74, **138**, 141
sulcus, 108
sweat gland, 88
sweating, 64, 81, 90, 105
Sydenham, Thomas, 147
synapse, 28, **30**, **33**, 36, **56**, 57, 60, **60**, 106
sympathetic chain, 106
syphilis, 76, 117, 121, 129

T
tabes dorsalis, 129
T-cell, 139
tear gland, 88, 106
teeth, **103**
temperature, 74, 90, 97
tendon, 65
tetanus, 66, 120
tetraethylammonium, 60
tetrodotoxin, 60
thalamus, 74, 106, 136, 140
thermoreceptor, **75**
thermo-regulation, 90, **91**, **92**
thiamine, 132
thirst, 90, 92, 93
thorax, 68, 88
thymus gland, 130
tongue, 41, 68, **74**
transcutaneous neural stimulation, 151
transmitter, **94**